D0891434

Situated Intervention

Inside Technology
edited by Wiebe E. Bijker, W. Bernard Carlson, and Trevor Pinch

Situated Intervention

Sociological Experiments in Health Care

Teun Zuiderent-Jerak

The MIT Press
Cambridge, Massachusetts
London, England

MIT Press books may be purchased at special quantity discounts for business or sales promotional use. For information, email special_sales@mitpress.mit.edu.

Set in Stone by the MIT Press. Printed and bound in the United States of America.

Library of Congress Cataloging-in-Publication Data

Zuiderent-Jerak, Teun, author.
Situated intervention : sociological experiments in health care / Teun Zuiderent-Jerak.
    p.   cm.—(Inside technology)
 Includes bibliographical references and index.
ISBN 978-0-262-02938-4 (hardcover : alk. paper)
I. Title. II. Series: Inside technology.
[DNLM: 1. Delivery of Health Care. 2. Sociology. 3. Quality of Health Care. W 84.1]
RA418
362.1—dc23
2015001897

10 9 8 7 6 5 4 3 2 1

~~for~~ with Sonja

Contents

Acknowledgments

Every scholarly work with one name on the cover performs the myth of single-authored scholarship. Although that myth may currently be well worth defending, acknowledgments are not the place to do so. If all books are networks, with relations and connections spreading in every direction, this is even more so for a book on situated intervention. Moreover, writing this book spanned more years than I wish to recall. That, too, makes it impossible to acknowledge all who contributed to its fruition. Nonetheless, I will attempt—and fail—to do so here.

I start with the care professionals, hospital administrators, policy makers, and patients who were much more than mere "research subjects." Given our inspiring mix of interests, loyalties, and productive betrayals, I'm particularly sorry that I cannot acknowledge some of the most important contributors by name, having promised them anonymity. I can only hope that all those who were involved in the research that led to chapters 1–3 will feel acknowledged through the small or large changes in their working lives or in their patients' lives that our shared involvement may have brought about. That would be the least I should hope for, given all the changes our interaction has enabled me to experience in my scholarly life.

Fortunately, the long-standing collaboration with the Atrium Medical Center is exempt from anonymity. I thank everyone there, and especially Nico van Weert, for being committed to quality improvement and to exploring in practice what that actually entails. Equally important for the research that led to chapter 4 was the collaboration with those involved in the Better Faster initiative—especially Marc Rouppe van der Voort, who is simply amazing at handling the logistics of health care, and Marije Stoffer, who turned individuals into a team.

There are many others without whom the book would never have been completed, but only one without whom it would not even have been started. Marc Berg crucially influenced my thinking about the materiality of intervention, about the role of STS scholars in relation to their fields, and about the possibility of doing health care differently. I am grateful for all that and much more. Extensive collaboration with Roland Bal shaped the book in important ways. His commitment to placing STS firmly in practices of health care governance, while staying part of both (or rather many) worlds, was crucial to the projects on which we collaborated and to many of the ideas developed herein. Ongoing conversations with Casper Bruun Jensen on intervention in STS were central to the overall argument and resonate especially in the conclusion. It was my enormous good fortune to have him as an enduring interlocutor. Stefan Timmermans generously gave extensive feedback on several drafts. The book benefited tremendously from his firm critique and his scholarly acumen.

The Research on IT in Healthcare Practice and Management section and later the Healthcare Governance section of the Institute of Health Policy and Management at Erasmus University Rotterdam provided crucial support and intellectual nourishment for many years. The Unit of Technology and Social Change (Tema T) at Linköping University is proving to be a wonderful new home, and I thank the Research Fellow program of the LiU Board for providing me ample academic freedom and time to complete the book. The work also benefited from scholarly presentation and discussion in several venues, including colloquia at Gothenburg University, at Virginia Tech, at the University of Copenhagen, and at the University of Twente. Although I had to postpone discussing this work till my very last event as coordinator of the Netherlands Graduate Research School of Science, Technology and Modern Culture (WTMC), my many discussions with participants and speakers were great sources of inspiration, for which I am deeply grateful.

I thank Geof Bowker for lovely conversations in which Serres, intervention, and spirituality share an equal place. Mike Lynch was a constant source of inspiring takes on intervention and scholarship , especially there where we ultimately draw slightly different conclusions. I thank Jessica Mesman for nearly two decades of support and inspiration. Gary Downey provided much support and stimulation for this work, both through dialogue and by co-editing (with Joe Dumit) a volume in which an inspiringly wide range of scholars addressed the topic of intervention.

The work benefited greatly from conversations with and feedback from Ingemar Bohlin, Huub Dijstelbloem, Steve Epstein, Lena Eriksson, Kor Grit, Willem Halffman, Hans Harbers, David Hess, Randi Markussen, Brian Martin, Morten Sager, Carsten Timmermann, Brit Ross Winthereik, and Paul Wouters. I thank Emilie Gomart for advising me to book "Appointments with Foucault, Location: Library" when "urgent" tasks in projects begin to take up most of my calendar space. Chapter 5 grew from a stimulating multidisciplinary collaboration with Anna Nieboer, Annemiek Stoopendaal, and Mathilde Strating. I thank them for the experience.

I am grateful to Aventis Behring, to an anonymous university hospital, to the Dutch Ministry of Health (through the Better Faster program), to the Netherlands Organisation for Health Research and Development (grant 53430001), and to the Scientific Council for Government Policy (a grant from the Market, State and Society project) for financial support. Ragini Werner of NEEDSer and Paul Bethge at the MIT Press provided excellent editorial support.

Portions of the book draw upon earlier articles, notably Zuiderent-Jerak 2007, 2009, 2010, Zuiderent-Jerak and Jensen 2007, Zuiderent-Jerak et al. 2009, Zuiderent-Jerak et al. 2012, and Zuiderent-Jerak et al. 2015. I am grateful to the publishers for permission to draw upon those articles.

Finally, I thank the person who comes first in so many ways. Sonja Jerak-Zuiderent, I keep on being amazed by the wonderful intertwinement of our personal, spiritual, and professional lives. I could not dedicate this book to you, for it is already ours.

Introduction: Exploring Intervention in the Social Sciences

The philosophers have only interpreted the world in various ways. The point, however, is to change it.

—Karl Marx, 1845

Whoever lacks the capacity to put on blinders, so to speak, and to come up to the idea that the fate of his soul depends upon whether or not he makes the correct conjecture at this passage of this manuscript may as well stay away from science.

—Max Weber, 1918

If you want to truly understand something, try to change it.

—Kurt Lewin, 1951

Dr. Maarten Pols is staring at a spreadsheet with a puzzled look on his face. The file contains an overview of clinical interventions performed on patients with colon cancer. To his surprise, he notices that he and his fellow gastroenterologists are not the only ones who regularly carry out colonoscopies to diagnose such patients. Surgical oncologists often repeat the procedure, using a diagnostic tool that causes discomfort for the patient, increases the risk of infection, and generates extra costs for the hospital. Gastroenterologists deem the tool outdated.

Dr. Pols[1] turns to Dr. Jan Roijers, the surgical oncologist present at this meeting devoted to improving the quality of internal medicine, and asks "If I have already established that it's bad news, why do the whole thing over again with a static scope?" He seems about to add "as if my examining patients once, with a flexible purging scope, isn't bad enough."

Dr. Roijers replies "If you and your colleagues didn't just tell us it's bad news, but assessed the exact tumor location, we wouldn't need to! But after discovering a few times during surgery that a patient should have had radiation therapy before the resection, we started taking our own measures." Dr. Roijers explains that this form of cancer stops being colon carcinoma when the tumor is located in the last 12–15 centimeters of the large intestine. In that case it is rectum carcinoma. Whereas colon carcinoma needs swift resection, mortality for rectum carcinoma is substantially reduced by radiation therapy before resection. Dr. Roijers is astonished that Dr. Pols was unaware of the importance of this distinction.

To avoid the possibility that in the future diagnostics will be carried out more than once, the doctors agree that the gastroenterologists will note the tumor's location more precisely. Veronica Vendeloo, a manager responsible for quality in internal medicine, agrees to monitor this change by providing regular updates of the spreadsheet and reporting to the improvement team as soon as double diagnostics reappear. Cluster manager Rob Timmer says he and one of the hospital's directors will present the change during upcoming contract negotiations with a leading insurance company. He hopes that showing how the hospital is reducing disorganization and waste will put him in a good position to contract other price increases that are really needed to improve quality.

Later that day, at a meeting devoted to improving the quality of surgery, Dr. Hans Brakema is discussing ways to reduce waiting times for his surgery hours. A week ago, I had looked at the types of visits that fill up his clinic. Now I asked him whether he really needed to conduct follow-ups on all patients having had small elective procedures. To my mind, such patients are generally happy that their minor discomfort has been fixed and often feel little need to pay another hospital visit, entailing taking time off from work or perhaps arranging for child care. Dr. Brakema responds emotionally: "It would be truly unethical if I plunged a knife into someone's body and never shook their hand afterwards!"

Ingrid Joosen, the quality manager at the meeting, suggests that rather than discussing ethical principles we should match the entries in the outpatient and surgery modules of the hospital information system, to find out how often the surgeon doing the follow-up is actually the one who operated. This proposal is not quite as innocent as it seems, because she knows that the surgeons have begun to use an internal division of labor that is at variance from the professional ethics they espouse. Some surgeons were simply far more efficient in the operating theater; others were better at running surgery hours—a fact not ignored when they faced pressure from hospital management and insurance companies to reduce exorbitant waiting times.

With help from the IT department, Ingrid Joosen produced the figures that we analyzed at the next meeting. It turns out that no more than 5 percent of all operated patients are seen during follow-up by the operating surgeon. We discuss how freeing space in his surgery hours would allow Dr. Brakema to stick to his professional ethics for at least some patients in oncology—for example, those whom the operating surgeon should personally inform about the level of metastasis found and how far a tumor has grown into the surrounding organs. At *present, a potentially laudable normative principle threatens the knife-plunging/ hand-shaking match for patients undergoing such complex procedures. We therefore decide to try nurse-led follow-up for small elective procedures. A nurse will call a patient the day after surgery and will go through a pre-defined checklist of complications. If all seems fine, the patient will see the surgeon for follow-up only if he or she wants to. For more complex procedures, patients will still be booked automatically for follow-up, always with the operating surgeon. Alma Heger, the manager of the outpatient clinic, will instruct the doctors' assistants who will make the appointments, and Ingrid Joosen will ask the IT department to set up an indicator measuring the match between operating surgeons and follow-up surgeons and send the results to Dr. Brakema each month.*

This book considers the question of how the direct involvement of social scientists in the practices they study can lead to the production of interesting sociological knowledge. The book draws together two activities that are often seen as belonging to different realms: intervening in practices and furthering scholarly understanding of them. The common separation of these domains stems in part from disciplinary self-understandings within sociology that are largely shaped by debates on the need for detached sociological scholarship or its mirror image of engaged social science.[2] Both sides in the debate draw on the problematic idea that knowing and acting are separate entities (Dewey 1929); they differ only as to which side of this dichotomy they privilege.

Within such a scholarly self-understanding, research that intervenes not with the primary aim of changing practice on the basis of sociological insight, but instead in order to *produce* sociological knowledge, is easily qualified as non-research. This consequence has regularly been made clear to me in the past ten years. When I submitted an article on intervening in the organization of a university hospital to learn more about the dynamics between standardization and patient-centered care, a reviewer for a leading medical sociological journal wrote: "This paper is a scholarly extension of what was in essence a clear-cut applied health services problem. ... The project was not conceived or executed as a research project and the result seems akin to salvage writing." The editor agreed, and the paper was rejected. Apparently, intervening in medical practice didn't qualify as doing sociological research.

Often, other actors in health-care-improvement settings are not averse to such divisions between knowing and acting. Once, at a meeting of managers and organizational advisors in a process-redesign project, I observed how we seemed to be coming up with a kind of standardization different from the one usually invoked in such projects, and this reconceptualiza-tion could help us think differently about the further redesign of care pro-cesses. One of the consultants challenged me: "But what we're doing here is applied science, isn't it?" When I failed to produce an instant coherent response to his rhetorical question, he continued: "Well, either we're doing basic science, or we're doing applied science, so this must be the latter." His message was "We're acting here, so please stop this superfluous think-ing." Besides making me wonder what "basic sociology of standardization in health care" would look like—probably something concerning a lab with gray OncoMice™ as patients, albinos as care professionals in their white coats and rats (why not?) as managers, acting out purely social relations in a model of a redesigned pathway—I found these events particularly telling because they showed the high level of agreement between academic soci-ologists and organizational advisors on their division of labor.

In this agreement on who is doing the knowing and who is doing the doing, being a member of a quality-improvement team (such as the ones described above) obviously has little to do with sociology. Intervening in the organization of hospital care is fine as quality improvement, but cannot be a valid scholarly approach to the sociological study of patient-centered care, patient safety, standardization, and health care markets. Yet, as I hope to show in this book, there are two main reasons why such interventions in health care practices may make for interesting practices of sociological inquiry.

The first reason is that, in contrast with what is assumed in the images of objective or basic science invoked by the reviewer and the consultant, philosophers of science such as Ian Hacking (1983) have argued that natu-ral sciences benefited tremendously from broadening their scholarly mode from *theorizing about the world* to *intervening through experiments*. Adhering to an objectivist theorizing image of scholarship in sociology therefore risks losing a mode of knowledge production that has proved highly produc-tive in the natural sciences. Could the sociology of health care markets benefit from a study of the intersection of colonoscopies with fixed scopes, patient safety and suffering, inter-professional coordination, cost reduc-tion, and insurer contracts? Couldn't such a study help us to learn about market ecologies in which competition and professional quality are not necessarily sociological antonyms (chapter 4)? And could I have learned all this without becoming the leader of a national quality-improvement project in which one of my roles was to develop spreadsheets and mea-surement instruments that would precisely articulate which interventions different professionals carried out at various times? In short, could there be

something to gain *in terms of sociological realism* by letting go of both scholarly objectivism and engaged sociology?

The second reason is that experimental interventions may prove relevant to discussions of the normativity of sociological research practices.
Such debates tend to be dominated by a dual fear: on the one hand a fear of
over-involvement and loss of epistemic distance and sociological identity,
and on the other hand a fear of over-detachment and failure to address the
issues that should really matter to us. Experimental intervening does not
operate from a detached scholarly position, nor does it aim at implementing
a pre-set normative agenda. In a similar vein to the *experimental production
of knowledge*, which assumes neither freely theorizing scholars nor applied
scientists who implement what is already known, scholarly intervention
allows for the *experimental production of normativity* which is a normative
stance presuming that scholars are far from detached but may still be surprised by the normative outcomes of experimental interactions. Before we
wanted to test and manipulate this normativity in the experimental setting
of a project to improve surgical care, neither Dr. Brakema nor I knew that in
our normative commitments to follow-up after surgery we failed to make
a distinction between different types of oncological or elective surgery. As
Susan Leigh Star says (1995, p. 25), "we can't know about the consequences
of including ourselves in the analysis until we try." Given that an increasing number of sociologically oriented scholars are trying to do just that—
include themselves in the practices they study and analyze—intervening
in practices as diverse as improving the quality of health care, (workplace)
ICT design, evidence production in forensic pathology, or scientific laboratory work,[3] I hope, in this book, to help articulate the emerging scholarly
practice of intervening to produce sociological knowledge and normativity,
and thereby reclaim the notion of intervention from static understandings
of objectivity and ethics.

Scholars, Fields, and Their Fraught Relations

The question of how social scientists relate to the actors they study is a
fundamental soul-searching topic in many academic disciplines. This discussion goes back at least to Karl Marx, who famously claimed that the
scholarly role is not to understand the world but to change it (1845), and
to Max Weber, who, in contrast, argued in *Science as a Vocation* (1918–19)
that the academic life calls for a position that voluntarily blinds itself to
all kinds of utilitarian concerns and political demands. These contrasts
regularly figure in debates on the societal role of academics in the popular

media. Here is an example from a 2004 *New York Times* op-ed piece by Stanley Fish: "Marx famously said that our job is not to interpret the world, but to change it. In the academy, however, it is exactly the reverse: our job is not to change the world, but to interpret it."[4]

Though it is somewhat ironic that Marx's critique of interpreting philosophers gets turned into a claim for philosophical interpretation, such calls for a distanced social science become all the more vigorous when the organization of scientific work seems to be moving in the opposite direction. With the shift toward project-based funding of scholarly work, "knowledge translation" sections of grant proposals increasingly require scholars to spell out the practical utility of research findings well in advance of a study, no matter how explorative the proposed scholarship may be. Furthermore, relatively new scientific fields such as Action Research, Computer-Supported Cooperative Work, and Participatory Design, and even younger fields such as Experience-Based Design (Bate and Robert 2007), Workplace Studies (Luff, Hindmarsh, and Heath 2000), and Corporate Ethnography (Cefkin 2009), are based on the notion that sociological understandings of the complexity of practices are useful for their improvement. This can easily make it seem as if the contributions scholars make to their fields are largely dependent on their willingness to contribute. Even medical historians, who until recently considered themselves to be relatively far removed from concerns about practical usefulness, find themselves having to live up to calls from funders and colleagues that they have a positive "impact" on the practices they study (Smith 2011). Across the wide range of social sciences and humanities, the calls for both distanced and involved scholarship are becoming increasingly loud.

In response, those who plead for social sciences to influence their fields are often making a moral argument for the importance of coming to an *engaged* scholarly practice (van de Ven 2007; Seifer 2010). This does not merely relate to the Marxist position of actualizing a political position through scholarly work, nor is it directly subject to Weber's argument that "the prophet and the demagogue do not belong on the academic platform" (1918–19, p. 146). Engagement is regularly presented as a strategy to overcome precisely the dualism of the objectivist and critical modes of scholarly work and produce scholarship that is both rigorous and relevant. Whereas objectivism starts from the premise that science requires a moral prescriptive to be objective, critical theory has specialized in arguing that such objectivism is epistemologically defunct. Deconstructing scientific truth claims and objectivism is, however, no longer the privileged hunting ground of critical theorists; it has become a substantial industry that finds its most influential patrons in CEOs of oil companies and airlines. Consequently, critical theory is subjected to a "critique of critique," the argument being that merely critiquing objectivism for its simplified epistemological realism has become risky now that the "truth" of climate change, for example, is strongly contested by economically motivated actors—which leaves critical theorists with strange bedfellows.[5]

Proposing an engaged social science as an alternative to critique claims to provide a way out of this stalemate of objectivism versus critique by moving "beyond" epistemological clashes. This solution may, however, replace scientific objectivism with normative positions for which it is largely unclear how the displayed engagements relate to the scholarly work at hand. A weak connection between engagement and scholarship raises the question whether engagement is not simply activism combined with scientific authority and "rigorous methodology," which would be a return to the form of objectivism that critical theory set out to challenge in the first place. As Michael Lynch says of this tension (2009, p. 103), "the move 'beyond' criticism or relativism tends to replace the discredited objectivism with platforms of epistemic privilege that function in a similar way." In such cases, engaged scholarship that combines normative positions with the rhetorical authority of scholarly work in fact reverts to objectified (or at least epistemologically privileged) normativity, which is ironic in the light of the original epistemic critiques. It risks ending up in a position that combines the worst of both scholarly worlds: simplified objectivism and sentimental normativity. Pleas for engaged scholarship may therefore once again cause friction with the vocation of social scientists, albeit a friction that is diametrically opposed to the problem Weber proposes. Whereas Weber states that "in the lecture-rooms of the university no other virtue holds but plain intellectual integrity" (1918–19, pp. 155–156), which for him means limiting scholarly work to "self-clarification and knowledge of interrelated facts" (ibid., 152), the possibility that arises when social scientists move "beyond" criticism toward engagement is that social scientists may revert to the very aura of intellectual integrity that critical theory initially set out to challenge. Though recent calls for engaged scholarship seem sympathetic at first and often resonate with the personal concerns of social scientists, they quickly strike at the heart of scholarly self-definitions.

Under-Problematizing Engagement

Engagement is obviously not a problematic notion for all actors. The idea that engagement needs problematization is deeply foreign to those who are not concerned with questioning existing agendas or who do not question epistemic realism. Besides those who set those very agendas, such as research funders, I see two groups of actors who tend to under-problematize engaged scholarship. The first group consists of scholars who adopt problem definitions pre-set by the actors they engage with; the second consists of organizational consultants. These two groups are relevant for debates on the relations between social scientists and their fields, as these actors are regularly encountered by sociologists who become involved in changing the practices they study.

Researchers who do not question epistemic realism typically are committed to contributing knowledge to pre-set problem definitions, rather than taking their research to be about unpacking such definitions and exploring the action repertoires such definitions imply. This work is often conceptualized in terms of finding "factors" and "barriers" that facilitate or hamper organizational or systems change, and these approaches form mainstream scholarship in fields such as Information Systems Research, Innovation Studies, and Health Services Research. Researchers in these fields may address issues of a certain normative weight, such as barriers to transitions toward sustainable energy, the lack of implementation of ICT in public sectors, and insufficient use of patient-safety tools, and may suggest that their work adds an "evidence base" to addressing social issues. This type of research deploys a narrow definition of the "usefulness" of scholarly work that typically produces a legitimacy problem for those scholars with a scholarly attachment to complicating underlying assumptions and addressing issues other than those defined by policy makers. The engagement is toward problem definitions as set by one group of actors (generally fairly influential ones); it runs into problems only when other actors are encountered who do not share this problem definition. Even so, these others are typically defined as a risk factor or an organizational barrier to a privileged change initiative.

While observing a national meeting on improving ways of preventing elderly patients from falling, I attended a plenary talk by a researcher from the National Prevalence Measurement of Care Problems. He presented the facts and figures on falls and emphasized the importance of implementing proven interventions, such as protective hip shorts, that prevent injury when aged adults fall. After the talk, a care professional came up to him and told him quite a different story about these shorts. She had found them to be quite dangerous, especially on psychogeriatric wards. She told him that although the shorts may have been tested on groups of clients not suffering from dementia who fell while wearing them properly, the investigators had failed to realize that people in psychogeriatric wards often fall *because* they are wearing the shorts—or, rather, not quite wearing them. When clients go to the toilet, she said, they often get confused when they want to get up and find they are wearing a very unusual item of clothing. They have forgotten why they are supposed to be wearing the shorts, and they cannot fall back on a lifetime routine for putting the shorts back on. Consequently, they often get off the toilet with their trousers and underpants draped around their ankles and, not surprisingly, tend to fall, often onto unprotected hips. On hearing about this, the researcher didn't even blink, and I was struck by how little the story affected him. The problem definition, the evidence of proven interventions, and his commitment to reducing falls through implementing proven interventions seemed barely challenged by the complexities of fall-prevention practices.

As I noted above, the second group that tends to under-problematize engaged scholarship consists of organizational consultants. Such consultants are ubiquitous in Western hospitals. In the course of my research I have had many interactions like the one described above. When I tell the consultants about my work on intervention as a mode of sociology, they typically state that they "intervene all the time" in the health care practices we are both involved in. The difference between consultancy and sociology is becoming even more confused because sociologists are increasingly "hired in," sometimes at rates not all that different from consultants' fees.[6] The distinctions are blurred even more because consultancy companies are increasingly employing junior consultants with part-time appointments in academic departments of business or management schools, combining their employees' aspirations for the academic credits of a PhD with their own interest in researching the complex issues they deal with daily. However, as Gary Downey and Juan Lucena helpfully clarify (1997, p. 120), an important aspect of *sociological or anthropological* hiring in practices is "making visible modes of theorizing that are otherwise hidden, thus possibly legitimizing alternate perspectives ... rooted in the field itself." This points to the importance of the scholarly aim that sets research problematizing engagement apart from research or consultancy that accepts the problem definitions encountered. The research Downey and Lucena refer to is about *reconfiguring the problem space* that dominates a certain practice rather than about providing evidence or solutions for *pre-defined* problem spaces. Of course, these boundaries—and the boundary work I am doing here—are contested. Surely there is interesting consultancy work that comes quite close to such a definition of its practice, and social-science research that aims to problematize policy assumptions but fails to do so in an interesting manner. These differences do, however, point to a distinction in the central focus of these modes of relating to the field.

In this sense, I see three practices that are somehow related to social scientists in which 'engagement' is not a problematic term. First, there is scholarly work that pursues a normative or political aim without specifying how this aim relates to their research practice, and risks tapping into epistemic authority for mundane normative claims. Second, some scholars are pursuing agendas set by other actors and trying to provide an evidence base for what works to achieve policy aims. Third, there are organizational consultants who act with, or rather for, the fields that employ them. These three positions are unlikely to be positions that more reflexively oriented social scientists envision for themselves; they are, rather, precisely the kinds of roles that medical sociologists have long tried to avoid in debates about how they relate to their fields. Such debates, which have a substantial history in medical sociology, have gained pertinence as a result of the combination of an increased focus on "knowledge translation" in the funding of social science and claims for engaged scholarship in response to the problems of critique. This has been going on for decades and is part of what Downey and Dumit (1997, p. 10) call "a fundamental change taking place in the academy itself."[7] The situation social scientists find themselves in today may, therefore, benefit from revisiting these long-standing debates about the tension between societal effects and scholarly aims.

Taking Sides in, or with, Sociology

In the late 1960s, several sociologists discussed the role of social scientists in relation to their fields, focusing on how social scientists were implicated in the study of "social problems." Because postwar sociology (especially that of the Second Chicago School of Sociology[8]) was intertwined with the study of urbanization,[9] their studies focused on societal issues encountered in housing projects in the early 1950s, and on related broader questions about what it takes to become a drug user, a psychiatric patient, or some other sort of outsider to society. In the sociology of deviance, sociologists analyzed the interactive process by which this outsider status was ascribed and obtained. In doing so they moved away from the commonly held idea that deviance was a quality inherent in individuals of a certain type, and that societal action and rectification were called for. They focused on meaning-making in sociological groups that William Isaac Thomas, one of the main contributors to the First Chicago School of sociological thought, characterized as "social wholes" (1914)—groups that Anselm Strauss later conceptualized as "social worlds" (1978). As Adele Clark and Susan Leigh Star note (2008, p. 115), some sociologists of the Second Chicago School began combining a "traditional focus on (1) meanings/discourse as related to ethnicity and neighborhood, and (2) the search for identity in the forms of work, practice, and memory." "This," Clark and Star continue, "resulted in a sociology that was both material *and* symbolic, interactive, processual, and structural." Work in symbolic interactionism caused tensions for sociologists who wondered whether their scholarship would serve "deviant communities" by showing that deviance was a label that could be challenged once societal norms were called into question or whether it would benefit research funders who assumed these communities to be the cause of societal troubles. Scholars struggled with their commitments to the cause of helping the "socially indigent" and with the risk that their studies would justify prevailing labeling practices. Lee Rainwater and David Pittman described their struggle this way (1967, p. 361): "If one describes in full and honest detail behavior which the public will regard as immoral, degraded, deviant, and criminal, will not the effect be to damage the very people we hope our study will eventually help?"

Despite these troubles, the substantial societal problems in the housing projects made a more detached sociological position an unattractive option to many. The segmentation of a scholarly vocation—professionally separated from personal affection—was fiercely criticized by many, including John Seeley, who, in direct reference to Weber, wrote:

[O]ne's profession, one's calling, vocation, *Beruf*, if it calls at all and so is a profession, calls out and calls upon all else, organizes, dominates, structures and gives point to all else. … Disjuncture, then, between professional and personal ethic bespeaks the institution of that alienation from the world which would imply a poor professional and a poor profession, or from the person which entails an impoverished professional and an impoverished self. (1967, p. 383)

This conceptualization of the sociological profession resulted in a debate on how sociologists could relate to their fields *without* pretending that their human concerns had nothing to do with their scholarly vocation. Seeley was most evidently radical when he suggested that the role of scholarship was *making* rather than *taking* problems, and that made problems had to be based on an ethical stance. Consequently, for Seeley, sociologists should "know in acceptable fullness not only where we want to go—or want society to go—but how we want it to get there, and how the criticism is to function in the getting of it there" (ibid., p. 387). Seeley justified this proposal by drawing an analogy to medical work and malpractice. As in medicine, it would be "negligent (i.e., morally reprehensible as well as technically

inept) to prescribe without knowledge of certain kinds, and in certain cases
... would establish the fact of criminality, legally, and the basis for professional penalties, socially, and justified serious adversion, morally" (ibid.).
Sociologists doing research on social problems without a firm ethical base
would be "like a collection of mad doctors" (ibid., p. 388). I will return to
this medical analogy later in this introduction, but for now it suffices to
note that proposing an ethical base for scholarly action has been and is
repeated persistently over time, despite the problems of combining ethical strategies with the epistemic authority that sociologists in the 1960s
would usually reserve for the top dogs they criticized rather than for the
underprivileged they wished to side with. Some problems that follow from
this stance become strikingly clear when Seeley proposes that in order to
establish this ethical base he wishes to "gather out a company" of those
agreeing with his analysis, and "explore for a common consent in those
large principles that have seemed to many to be the meeting ground for all
humane and reasonable men, and for others to have the nature and status
of 'natural law'" (ibid.). In this manner the sociology of deviance has led
Seeley into a rather absolutist—even "natural"—normativity. Despite the
"reasonable" ethics Seeley hopes for, its absolutism would inevitably produce its own deviances, which would present sociologists with the dilemma
whether to side with deviants or to authoritatively stick to their own (or
"nature's") moral order. Fortunately, a somewhat more ambivalent suggestion about the role of the social sciences is found in the debate between
Howard Becker and Alvin Gouldner.

In an influential yet widely misunderstood article titled "Whose side
are we on?" Becker acknowledges both the impossibility of a value-neu-
tral social science and the need to abstain from simplifying the normative
complexity of practices. The general interpretation of this article is that
Becker claims that, since value-neutrality is unattainable, sociology should
side explicitly with the underdog. He does indeed say that value-neutrality
is "imaginary" (1967, p. 239), and also that sociologists "usually take the
side of the underdog" (ibid., p. 244). But, crucially, he also states that sociologists ought "to make sure that, whatever point of view we take, our
research meets the standards of good scientific work, that our unavoidable
sympathies do not render our results invalid" (ibid., p. 246). To ensure that
sociologists' taking sides is not at odds with good scholarly work, Becker
introduces two related principles: first, sociologists should "avoid sentimentality," meaning that scholars should not shun finding out "what is
going on, if to know would be to violate some sympathy"; second, sociologists should study "impartially," meaning that sociological techniques

should be applied so that "a belief to which we are especially sympathetic could be proved untrue." According to Hammersley (2001, p. 99), Becker thus seems to argue both that "we cannot avoid taking sides and that we should avoid taking sides."

Furthermore, Becker points out that there is a difference between taking sides and being accused of doing so. Accusations of sociologists' bias may be due precisely to their applying sociological theories impartially. The social systems studied have what Becker calls a "hierarchy of credibility," meaning that "people consider the source of any statement or perception, and discount those produced by lower-status people" (Star 1995, p. 1). Consequently, respectable groups have a greater right to define the way things really are than deviant groups. Thus, by giving equal credence to statements of outsiders and to those of responsible officials, impartial sociology of deviance may provoke the charge of bias. Becker also points out that, conversely, sociology that is less impartial because it takes a position in favor of the established order is far less likely to be accused of bias, because that position does not show disrespect for the prevailing hierarchy of credibility. Thus, Becker's argument is far more nuanced than a simplified plea for pursuing a political position of empowering underdogs through scholarship. Becker argues for a sociology that tends to favor underdog positions, but is careful to avoid sentimentality about such attachments, while realizing that accusations of bias are more likely if it follows the dictum of impartiality instead of uncritically taking sides with prevailing hierarchies of credibility. Becker therefore closes his article with a note on sociological strategy:

We take sides as our personal and political commitments dictate, use our theoretical and technical resources to avoid the distortions that might introduce into our work, limit our conclusions carefully, recognize the hierarchy of credibility for what it is, and field as best as we can the accusations and doubts that will surely be our fate. (Becker 1967, p. 247)

This combination of taking sides, allowing for surprising normativities through avoiding sentimentality, facing the accusations of bias that follow from impartiality, and (importantly) living with the doubt this generates can hardly be seen as a flat-out plea for partisan scholarship. Yet that is exactly what Becker has both been praised and criticized for.

In a 1968 article titled "The sociologist as partisan," Alvin Gouldner states that sociology comes "to confess its own captivity" and expresses the fear that "the once glib acceptance of a value-free doctrine is about to be superseded by a new but no less glib rejection of it" (p. 103). This nicely captures the dual fear that underlies much of the debate on the role of the social sciences in relation to their fields: sociologists are either too detached or too involved. This fear seems to stem from defining the problem of sociology as finding a position between two ends of a scale with the mutually exclusive and equally unattractive poles of partisanship and objectivity. According to Gouldner, at one end of the scale sociology's recent "orientation to the underworld" comes with a partisanship that, referring to Marxist ideologies, "has become the equivalent of the proletarian identifications felt by some intellectuals during the 1930s" (ibid., p. 104). At the other end, we find the solution of compartmentalizing social science and morality. "Weber fantasies [sic] a solution in which facts and values will each be preserved in watertight compartments," Gouldner notes, pointing out that "the pursuit of 'truth for its own sake' is always a tacit quest for something more than the truth, for other values that may have been obscured, denied, and perhaps even forbidden, and some of which are expressed in the quest for 'objectivity'" (ibid., pp. 115–116).

That Gouldner places Becker at the end of the scale he calls "empty-headed partisanship" (ibid., p. 116) is the most extreme version of the radical reading of Becker's argument.[10] It seems peculiar in view of the ambiguities in Becker's article,[11] and it hardly seems fair to assert that Becker's warning against sentimentality about personal commitments equals "a myth that holds it possible to have a sentiment-free commitment" (ibid., p. 105). Yet Gouldner does raise interesting questions. If simple-minded side-taking is such an unwelcome option, are there any good *scholarly* reasons to conduct research from the underdog standpoint? Is there any chance that following the political commitments of many scholars would make them better *sociologists*? Gouldner sees two advantages in doing so: first, sociologists would be able to learn something about social worlds they themselves and many others know little or nothing about; second, it would give sociologists a new perspective on worlds that they and others assumed they knew a good deal about. Though his dual fear stops Gouldner from working out the answer to this question in more detail, so that it stays at the level of good research as producing more (and perhaps more interesting) knowledge, it is interesting that he tries to realign scholarly and personal commitments.

Gouldner's radical reading of Becker is, however, particularly illustrative of how discussions of the role of social sciences in relation to their fields lead either to polarized debates that juxtapose Marx and Weber or to more nuanced contributions that attract remarkably little attention.[12] Such is the case for this early debate, but polarization has continued to dominate discussions over the years,[13] despite marginalized claims to open these matters up for empirical enquiry (Denzin 1968).

One of the more recent manifestations of sociological soul-searching that proposes a split between scholarly engagement and academic professionalism is Michael Burawoy's call for "public sociology." In his influential 2004 presidential address to the American Sociological Association, Burawoy expressed concern that sociology had become caught in a wave of progress that made it shed its "original passion for social justice, economic equality, human rights, sustainable environment, political freedom or simply a better world" (2005, p. 5). "If our predecessors set out to change the world," Burawoy says, implicitly referencing Marx, "we have too often ended up conserving it." (ibid.) To alleviate this loss, Burawoy proposes dividing sociological labor into professional, critical, policy, and public sociology, of which the extremes of detachment and involvement—professional and public sociology—are to be seen as complementary:

We have spent a century building professional knowledge, translating common sense into science, so that now, we are more than ready to embark on a systematic back-translation, taking knowledge back to those where it came from, making public issues out of private troubles, and thus regenerating sociology's moral fiber. Herein lies the promise and challenge of public sociology, the complement and not the negation of professional sociology. (ibid.)

Reviewing the extensive discussion that this call sparked is beyond the scope of this book, but a few things are noteworthy in the light of the history of such debates.

First, the complementary nature of the divided labor *itself* shows that the entire argument is once again structured around a firm separation of sociological *knowing* and sociological *acting*. The first is represented by professional (and critical) sociology focused on developing scholarly legitimacy through scientific expertise (ibid., p. 10). The second is a part of public (and policy) sociology that is concerned mainly with seeking out, engaging, and producing publics that can be helped by such sociological knowledge. As a consequence of this split, many of the responses are fully fed by the double fear this division of labor provokes. The driving force, for Burawoy, is clearly the fear of being too detached. Professional detachment without public sociology results in the failure of sociologists to safeguard society and even humanity that Burawoy sees as "beleaguered by the encroachment of markets and states" (ibid., p. 4). Some publications endorse this fear—sometimes with explicit reference to the Marxist and Weberian histories, as in Charles Derber's call for "public sociology as a vocation" in Burawoy et al.

2004. The critics quickly slide into the opposite fear of being too involved. They argue that sociological knowledge is not good enough yet, or that embarking upon public sociology will so reduce the legitimacy of the discipline that none of its statements will be heard. Arthur Stinchcombe, for example, argues that "we must tend to our job of getting enough truth of the kind than can bear on the future [and] that is so difficult that we should not be distracted much by contributing to public discourse" (2007, p. 135).[14] Meanwhile, Douglas Massey expresses concern that "a reputation for impartiality and objectivity greatly enhances the value of the statements that the [American Sociological] association *does* choose to make on questions of public import [and] provides sociologists with a means to build professional respect and scientific prestige and, hence, the legitimacy to weigh in on debates as individuals" (2007, pp. 147–148).

Second, it is striking that, whereas Gouldner is referenced in the original presidential address, Becker's "Whose side are we on?" is not merely left out of Burawoy's argument, it is not even referenced in any of the published symposia in *Social Problems* (February 2004), *Social Forces* (June 2004), and *Critical Sociology* (May 2005), or in its most influential edited volume (Clawson et al. 2007). And even Gouldner is invoked (under Burawoy's heading THESIS XI: SOCIOLOGIST AS PARTISAN) to argue that "the standpoint of sociology is civil society and the defense of the social" and that "in times of market tyranny and state despotism, sociology—and in particular its public face—defends the interest of humanity" (Burawoy 2005, p. 24). Thus, the debate on public sociology is not infomed by Becker's suggested principles of avoiding sentimentality and studying impartially, or by his warning that partiality is often a matter of ascription rather than of position, *or* by Gouldner's suggestion that there may be *professional scholarly* reasons to pursue political commitments. As a consequence, the split between academic credentials and personal concerns proliferates, as does sociologists' dually fearful relationship with the worlds they study.

Siding with Sociology or Medicine

Discussions of the relation of *medical* sociology to the field of medicine also have a long history, and have in fact been quite defining for the shift from *medical* sociology to the sociology of *health and illness* (Timmermans and Haas 2008). In one of the texts that established medical sociology as a field, Robert Straus distinguished between sociology *of* medicine and sociology *in* medicine, asserting that the former must be carried out at a distance from medicine and that the latter can be pursued in collaboration (1957, p. 203).

With the by now easily recognizable fear of being too engaged, Straus suggested that the two are incompatible and that sociology *in* medicine may jeopardize the sociologists' professional identity: "If the sociologist begins to talk like a physician, he may eventually come to act like a physician and even to think like a physician. If he sacrifices his identity as a sociologist, he loses the unique contribution he can make to medicine." (ibid., p. 204) Still, this contribution to medicine *was* an important aim for Straus, who spent most of his professional life working at a medical school. (See Straus 1999.) He therefore also expressed the other fear of being too detached: sticking to "pure sociology in the face of demands for interpretation (and there is need for pure sociology in medicine at the right time and place) will be misunderstood, ignored or rejected" (Straus 1957, p. 204).

Despite Straus's dual warning, it seems as if his colleagues initially picked up his first recommendation especially, to protect professional identity. As Stefan Timmermans and Steven Haas point out, the editors of early editions of the *Handbook of Medical Sociology* asserted that "there are no reasons for the development of unique or special theories in medical sociology" and that "medical sociology, like all sociology, is concerned with social relationships and social processes, and its theoretical base must of necessity be that of general sociology" (Freeman, Levine, and Reeder 1963, 1972, 1979, pp. 506, 476, 467). According to those editors, medical sociology was firmly about sociology, not medicine. According to Timmermans and Haas (2008, p. 661), they tried to shield the discipline from "evolving into an applied discipline, especially a social science subservient to clinical medicine." Margaret Gold strongly pointed out this risk in a paper titled "A crisis of identity: The case of medical sociology." Gold analyzes a series of publications in medical sociology and concludes that most studies are highly influenced by medical value assumptions and that funding structures make sociologists dependent on clinicians in collaborative research. She proposes "strengthening the identity of medical sociology *as* sociology" (1977, p. 166) to ward off the threat of the identity crisis that follows from a lack of professional autonomy. This selective reading of Straus's warning seems more recently to have resulted in a tendency that is quite opposite to what Gold noticed in the late 1970s. In their review of publications of the last decade in *Sociology of Health and Illness*, Timmermans and Haas note that "social scientists have become mainly interested in the experience, culture, and social structuring of illnesses while bracketing the biological bedrock of disease" (2008, p. 660). This development has brought sociology closer to an underdog medical sociology than Gold could have held possible and produces new tensions between medical sociologists and clinical practice.[15]

Annette Lawson reports on a medical professor at Stanford who advised students that "they might like to avoid the 'anti-medicine elective'[:] my course in Medical Sociology" (1991, p. 592). In line with Becker's hierarchy of credibility, such advice could stem from the way a high-status medical profession can downplay medical sociologists, which is the explanation Lawson seems to adopt when she writes that "if being on the side of the underdog has led to unbridled attacks on medicine (defined as doctors) then that has clearly operated against sociologists" (ibid.). If medical sociology fails to take the more substantive position that Timmermans and Haas propose, the distance between medicine and sociology may result in a medical sociology that would exclude "clinical endpoints" and thereby the "normative purpose of health care," because of which medical sociology becomes "clinically unanchored" by ignoring "what often matters most to patients and health care providers" (2008, p. 659).

This does not mean that there are no substantive *problems* with the proposed closer alignment of medical sociology to the fields it studies. For example, after Stefan Timmermans and Marc Berg said in the epilogue to their 2003 book *The Gold Standard* that the study of the improvement of quality and safety in health care provides refreshing opportunities for various strands of the social sciences to gain societal relevance, Casper Bruun Jensen responded that this would allow the patient-safety *agenda* to be set solely by existing institutions, such as the US Institute of Medicine, leaving medical sociologists no other option than to take "the critical stance" or to enter "a vibrant future, in which medical sociologists are reconfigured as system designers" (2008, p. 321). According to Jensen, this would confine medical sociologists to contributing to better design of systems with preset agendas, even when their research shows interesting complexities that problematize policy assumptions underlying such agendas.[16] Debates about the role and the identity of the social sciences are not merely professional turf wars over autonomy and accountability; they are substantive debates on crucial scholarly attachments. The idea that one is either committed to sociology or engaged with issues in the practices studied may preclude exactly what scholars have to add *sociologically* to these practices and what these practices have to offer for sociology.

From Engagement to Intervention

As discussions of the role and identity of social scientists reveal, the notion of "engaged social science research" presents scholars with questions about what to engage with and about how such engagements relate to prevailing scholarly aims. It also poses a legitimacy problem for scholars wanting to articulate their theoretical engagement in rethinking pre-defined problem definitions, who may be told that their work "risks being consigned to quietism or, worse, mere academic professionalism" (Lynch 2006, p. 820). The very term "engaged research" raises the question of what the social sciences could possibly be when they are *not* engaged.[17] In this book I explore modes of social science's involvement that do not suffer from these problems of engagement. I do so by focusing on a notion that is generally reserved for the practices that sociology studies: intervention.

According to the philosopher of science Ian Hacking, intervention is a crucial concept for analyzing what scientific practices entail. In his influential 1983 book *Representing and Intervening,* Hacking challenges the importance of theorizing, which often is seen as *the* dominant scientific style aimed at coming to a good representation of nature.[18] He devotes the second half of the book to the importance of various forms of experimental intervening in the sciences. Scientific theorizing, especially because of the undue attention it has received in the philosophy of science, is one of the reasons why debates on realism and relativism have become so fruitless.[19] "Realism," Star explains (1995, p. 9), "is the position that 'there really is a there out there, and it's true in some absolute sense." "Relativism," Star continues, "holds that truths are relative to a place, time, or person (often a historical situation or geographic/cultural location)." According to Hacking, a reappraisal of experimental intervening in scientific knowledge production is crucial for addressing the philosophical problems of realism more productively. "Engineering, not theorizing," Hacking writes near the end of his book (p. 274), "is the best proof of scientific realism about entities. My attack on scientific anti-realism is analogous to Marx's onslaught on the idealism of his day. Both say that the point is not to understand the world but to change it."

Whereas Marx has been quoted to legitimize pursuing *political* aims through engaged scholarly work, and (by Stanley Fish) to show that such aims do not suit epistemic attachments, Hacking invokes Marx to pursue the *epistemic* aim of coming to pragmatically reliable knowledge. Intervening is not *the result* of engagement or of theorizing; rather, it is a *conditio sine qua non* for coming to a form of knowledge that Hacking calls "uncontentious realism" (ibid., p. 131). This notion of realism does not assume that entities really do exist and that the sciences can describe them objectively, which caused so much confusion in earlier debates on the scholarly role; rather, it assumes that "reality has to do with causation and our notions of reality are formed from our abilities to change the world" (ibid., p. 146).

Hacking thereby makes clear that there may be reasons that have little to do with engagement for pursuing an academic strategy of intervention: scientists intervene to explore and produce robust forms of knowledge. In this sense, Hacking refers in an unusual way to Marx, and in fact seems to end up at a point that is generally ascribed to Kurt Lewin, who supposedly wrote that in order to truly understand something one should try to change it.[20]

In line with this more agential understanding of intervening as the production of reality, Hacking's understanding of experimental knowledge production is quite different from common-sense understandings of the scientific experiment. *Instantiae crucis* (or, as later rendered, "crucial experiments") are often depicted as a way to test two theories that have competing truth claims with the aim of providing the conclusive answer as to which theory is correct. Drawing on the writings of the seventeenth-century philosopher of science Francis Bacon, Hacking shows how this is *not* what Bacon has to say about experiments. For Bacon, *instantiae crucis* should be considered "fingerposts that are set up where roads part, to indicate the several directions" (Hacking 1983, p. 249). Experiments are therefore not devices with which to bring interpretation to an end, but rather devices with which to point to possible directions and their consequences, realizing that the fingerposts may well be misleading (ibid., p. 251). Experimentation, according to Hacking's reading of Bacon, is thus not a device for doing away with reflexivity, but rather a device for heightening it. Thus, whereas mainstream philosophy of science considers the experiment a controlled *demonstration device* to show that certain facts are "self-evident" (as Steve Shapin and Simon Schaffer argue in their 1985 book *Leviathan and the Air-Pump*), Bacon's understanding of the experiment was far more tentative and creative. In this sense, Bacon's ideas on scientific experimentation turn out to be much closer to current understandings of experimentation within the social sciences that emphasize its emerging improvised, surprising, generative side.[21]

Hacking's plea for the notion of experimental intervening to analyze what the natural sciences do is relevant to the present discussion of the role of the social sciences in relation to their fields. If scientific practices intervene for reasons other than societal engagement, I propose, the notion of experimental intervention may help to overcome social scientists' fear of either being too detached from normative concerns or being "merely useful" and co-opting with practice—the dual fear that is usually fanned when the quotation from Marx is employed critically or favorably. Interestingly, Hacking and others who point out the importance of experimental intervening for *understanding* how scientific knowledge production can be studied without getting stuck in naive notions of realism seldom explore the implications of their conclusions for scholarly practices in their *own* fields, be they philosophy of science or the social sciences and humanities at large. According to Hacking,[22] although 'intervening' is a crucial notion for studying the natural sciences, in his analysis it remains largely limited to the natural sciences, which implies that for other scientific practices the analogical-hypothetical style of reasoning—theorizing—remains largely unquestioned. This is somewhat ironic, not only in view of Hacking's sharp observation that "harm comes from a single-minded obsession with representation and thinking and theory, at the expense of intervention and action and experiment" (ibid., p. 131) but also because Hacking does in fact allude to the importance of intervention for the future of philosophy: "Natural science since the seventeenth century has been the adventure of the interlocking of representing and intervening. It is time that philosophy caught up to three centuries of our own past." (ibid., p. 146) In that sense, this book, by exploring the interlocking of representing and intervening in the social sciences, tries to do for sociology what Hacking proposes for philosophy.

Not only is this practice of reserving "intervention" for the sciences that are studied commonly encountered among philosophers of science; it is equally commonly encountered in medical sociology. In that scholarly domain, interventions are generally seen as clinical procedures carried out by health professionals, rather than as a mode of knowledge production for medical sociology. Medical, clinical, or surgical interventions belong to medicine and not to the sociology of health and illness. Since sociological interventions in health care practices form the empirical material in this book, working with the notion of interventionist scholarship is a dual attempt to relieve research practices of the moral weight of "engagement," simultaneously reclaiming some of the ideas about "where the action is" from the practices social scientists deal with.

Intervention can, of course, be seen as a crude notion, especially when mistakenly depicted as if it presupposes a contextual "outside" separate from a practice into which the intervention is "inserted," while the "outside" remains untouched and unchanged by the act. This critique defines intervention as "the idea of a one-way causation" and "the bringing forth of a completely new order through overt use of power" (Nickelsen 2009, pp. 10–11). Though etymologically the Latin meaning of *inter* (between) and *venīre* (to come) may indeed lead one to define intervention as a uni-directional action, in this book I stay closer to the ideas about intervening that Hacking explored for the sciences, and for which he continues to draw on seventeenth-century philosophy of science. According to Hacking (1983, p. 149), Francis Bacon "taught that not only must we observe nature in the raw, but that we must 'twist the lion's tail', that is, manipulate our world in order to learn its secrets." In that sense, revitalizing the notion of intervention for the *social* sciences could contribute to the "Back-to-Bacon movement" Hacking hopes to initiate. The involvement that follows from the explicit aim of changing a practice in order to learn from it, Hacking argues, has consequences for the proof that gets produced and, I would add, for scholars' resultant normative attachments. In this sense, intervention is diametrically opposed to implementation.

From Engagement as a Resource to the Topic of Situated Intervention

An important consequence of the shift from "engaged" to "intervening" social sciences is that sociologists no longer claim privileged access to a moral resource that justifies their engagement; rather, they unpack intervention as an empirical topic. This topic/resource distinction, which is central to ethnomethodology's program (Garfinkel 2002), was originally worked out in relation to the use of formal structures in sociological analyses. According to Harold Garfinkel and Harvey Sacks (1970, p. 337), "natural language serves persons doing sociology, laymen or professionals, as circumstances, as topics, and as resources of their inquiries furnishes to the technology of their inquiries and to their practical sociological reasoning *its* circumstances, *its* topics, and *its* resources."[23] This implies that, as Michael Lynch puts it (1993, pp. 148–149), the "intelligible theoretical position" is not found "'outside' the fields of practical action studied in sociology." When applied to social structures this means that, although the practices that produce and reproduce structures are topics of sociological analysis, *conceptions of* social structures should not be used as explanatory external resources.

The topic/resource distinction is usually deployed for the purpose of shifting the mode of analysis of the same concept, as in the case of "social structure." This is, however, somewhat problematic in relation to the notion of "engagement" since its very characteristic is that it draws on external resources. "Engagement" is therefore a particularly tricky notion for my aim for this book. Rather than apply the topic/resource distinction to the notion of engagement itself, I prefer to avoid altogether this notion that is so often employed *as a resource* and move on from engagement as a resource to the topic of intervention.[24] Applying the topic/resource distinction to "engagement" and "intervention" bypasses the dual fear and identity crises that interventionist social scientists otherwise incur, by relocating the question of normativity firmly *in* the practice of doing intervention. Whereas engaged social sciences tend to position normativity as part of the engagement resource to be drawn upon, interventionist social sciences locate normativity in the many attachments that actors in the field, including scholars, sort out in practice (Jensen 2007). This does not imply that social scientists' first fear of over-detachment need raise its head, but it does imply that their own attachments are neither completely pre-defined and based on partisanship nor valid only when justified by a scientific methodology.

Shifting from engagement as a resource to the topic of intervening means that interventions become situated. By this I mean, following Lucy Suchman, that interventions, rather than focus on actualizing an engaged agenda, should be part of "the context of particular, concrete circumstances" (1987, p. viii). As Suchman clarifies in response to some misreadings of her groundbreaking work on the relation between plans and situated actions, this does not imply that situated actions are merely reactive to the practice encountered or "synonymous with spontaneous or improvisational [actions]" (2007, p. 16). Nor should situatedness be interpreted as "involving a kind of erasure of context, as implying that action happens de novo, without reference to prior histories" (ibid.). It is worth reiterating these points here to prevent a similar misreading of situated intervention as entailing purely locally contingent experiments that are sociologically and normatively ahistorical. In contrast, situated intervention is a scholarly approach in which intervening aims at producing sociological knowledge by situating such interventions in sociologically unpacked normative complexities. My aim for this book is to contribute to the study of situated intervention as a topic in the social sciences.

Engagement and Situated Intervention in Science and Technology Studies

Though the role of the social sciences in relation to their fields is debated in many academic disciplines, in this book I focus on the contribution that the field of Science and Technology Studies (STS) can make to the larger discussion. Without essentializing STS (a young, dynamic, nomadic, interdisciplinary, and inherently incoherent field), I believe that many of the debates in this field provide great leverage when one is trying to pre-empt the two mirror images of simplified epistemic realism and normative standpoint absolutism. In this sense, drawing on the field of STS is helpful when one is conceptualizing the terrain that lies in between more "contentiously realist" streams in sociology that work with problem definitions set by influential actors and standpoint emancipatory fields such as participatory action research.[25] On the other hand, not all of this potential leverage has been fully deployed in STS to reflect on the issue of intervention, so the aim of this book allows me to both draw on and contribute to STS debates on the topic of intervention. I hope this makes my conceptualization relevant for scholars in the field, as well as for scholars facing similar questions in the social sciences and humanities at large.

Intervention has been a topic on the STS research agenda for several decades at least. STS shared its interest in demystifying science and technology by combining fieldwork and anti-positivism with the work of American symbolic interactionists (Star 1995, p. 6). One form this demystification took was the work of researchers in Edinburgh's "strong programme in the sociology of knowledge" in the 1970s. One of its tenets was that sociology should be "symmetrical in its style of explanation," meaning that "the same types of cause would explain, say, true and false beliefs" (Bloor 1976, p. 5). In the ensuing decades, STS researchers noticed that applying this principle to the study of technoscientific controversies entangled them in their objects of study in unforeseen ways. Marginalized actors in scientific disputes embraced STS analyses to such an extent that scholars felt captured by them. As a consequence, scholarly non-intervention seemed an impossibility, since "an epistemologically symmetrical analysis of a controversy is almost always more useful to the side with less scientific credibility or cognitive authority. In other words, epistemological symmetry often leads to social asymmetry or nonneutrality." (Scott, Richards, and Martin 1990, p. 490) Or, as Steve Woolgar noted about a decade earlier, "notwithstanding the declared intentions of the sociologist, the proffered alternative account will be heard as a comment on the adequacy of the original account" (1983, p. 254), and therefore, as David Hess noted (1997, p. 161), "the party with the lower credibility may seize a neutral account because it implicitly levels the playing field." Though the consequences of social scientists' being captured by those with lower credibility were different than earlier sociological experiences that faced challenges by credible actors, Becker's notion of hierarchies of credibility would have been helpful to make the experiences of Pam Scott, Evelleen Richards, and Brian Martin come as less of a surprise.[26] Since being captured *was* a surprise, it sparked the insight that the notion of the scientist as a detached observer of epistemic practices was not merely worthy of critique in the natural sciences; it equally created stimulating tensions for STS researchers studying technoscientific controversies.[27] Consecutive publications on this topic pointed out that intervention was not something that could be avoided, nor was it a problem as such; rather, repeating sociological debates, some STS researchers argue in these publications that the field should take positions, while others saw this situation as an empirical domain worth exploring[28] (cf. Blume 2000).

The notion of scholars as "captives" was developed in relation to the study of scientific controversies. Perhaps as an artifact of such controversial settings, it has been conceptualized as the aim of one homogenized party—this time the underdog instead of the establishment—to hold captive the scholar who was strengthening their cause.[29] These early studies focused on the "unintended consequences" of scholarly work and were not intentionally trying to intervene in the fields that captivated it, let alone carry out research that was commissioned to change a certain practice. Studies of controversies have been popular in STS, following from the assumption that sociological enquiry is ideally located in controversial events, since this is where the scholar gains insights into otherwise undisclosed mechanisms (Cambrosio and Limoges 1991; Rip 1986). As Michel Callon, Pierre Lascoumes, and Yannick Barthe put it (2009, p. 26), controversy "organizes the more complete investigation of possible states of the world." However, if we consider that controversies may produce *crucially different networks* than those one would encounter for more complex issues and multiple positions (Bal 1998; Halffman 2003; Mulkay, Potter, and Yearley 1983), this would have far-reaching consequences for a notion of intervention that draws heavily on controversial settings. And, as Brian Martin points out, there may be many cases in which the relationships between social scientists and other actors are nothing like the unidirectional experiences analyzed in the early 1990s, and therefore, 'capture' is "perhaps the wrong word since it connotes unwillingness on the part of the captured," and "'mutual enrolment' or 'joining forces' are more appropriate descriptions" (1996, p. 265). The question these alternative notions raise is, of course, "Joining forces with what or whom?"

The notion of "joining forces" again presumes to some extent that social scientists have to "take sides" with pre-defined parties. In the wake of claims that STS has depoliticized its "roots in activist struggles" (Martin 1993)[30] and its base in "radical social movements: radical science, feminism, women's health, civil rights, environmental justice, peace and so on" (Hess 1997, p. 157), the emergence of interventionist approaches is often positioned as a reply to the critique that constructivist studies provide "no grounds for making a decision about what course of action one ought to take" (Hess 2001, p. 236). This is the problem of what critics have called "the normative deficit of STS" (Keulartz et al. 2004, p. 12), or "the normative vacuum of STS" (Fuller 1999, p. 27). It comes down to the idea that this field is better suited to *studying* differences than to *making* a difference and that it "suffers from normative confusion, an incapacity to pronounce on whether it likes or dislikes what it so perspicuously sees" (ibid., pp. 27–28). Challenged by such criticism, Hess posits a "second generation" of ethnography-inspired STS researchers who tend "to be more oriented toward social problems (environmental, class, race, sex, sexuality and colonial)" (2001, p. 236). This move—highly similar to the partisanship Becker was accused of and to the idea that the social sciences can move "beyond" relativism by becoming "engaged," if only scholars cared to shift their orientation—seems to provide researchers with the normative purchase to "develop ways of intervening in their field sites as citizen-researchers and [make] their competence applicable to policy problems" (Hess 2001, p. 239). In this sense, Hess sees intervention as the analysis of how practices "might be *better* constructed, with the [criteria] of 'better' defined explicitly and their contestability openly acknowledged as both epistemological and political" (ibid., p. 240). Hereby, intervention becomes reattached to activism and social movements, to the Science and Society movement of the 1960s (Rose and Rose 1969), and to such related emancipatory initiatives as the Dutch (and, later, European) science shops of the 1970s and the 1980s (Wachelder 2003; Leydesdorff and Ward 2005). The normativity of STS research is hence relocated in the connection to its activist roots, much as partisanship was read into Becker's argument as a solution for an overly detached sociology. These ties between intervention and activism are further strengthened in a proposal for a "*rapprochement* … between the more academic and the more activist wings of STS" (Woodhouse et al. 2002, p. 297). In that proposal, Edward Woodhouse, David Hess, Steve Breyman, and Brian Martin reflect further upon the high value that many of the STS researchers they call "reconstructivist" ascribe to explicitly normative components of scholarly work, and connect their focus on intervention to grassroots issues and the democratization of the design of technologies.

This approach rejoins intervention and engagement as a resource, thereby also reintroducing the problems and ironies that face engaged scholarship. Taking the position of "citizen-researchers" risks reenacting normative standpoints rather than opening them up and preventing what Becker called "sentimentality." It thereby moves away from what Hess himself elsewhere calls "'good ethnographies' [that] frequently interrogate or complexify the taken-for-granted, such as common sense categories employed by social scientists, policy makers, activists and scientists" (2001, p. 239). Critical STS may therefore first re-instantiate and then critique the usual suspects, rather than empirically unpacking, complexifying, and re-situating normativities. This move could easily be seen as a typical case of one step forward and two steps back, in the light of the problems of the notion of "engaged" scholarship and the fact that it presumes that STS researchers have privileged "access to the 'larger picture' of social and institutional developments" (Jensen and Lauritsen 2005, pp. 67–68).

But just as there is a wide range of proposals to deal with these questions about the relation between social scientists and their fields, the rapprochement between activism and scholarly work is only one of the modes of intervention pursued in STS. An alternative follows by drawing lessons from how intervention is actually done in the practices that are sociologically studied. Studying how intervention is enacted in sciences that Hacking says have a three-century head start in analyzing the interlocking of representing and intervening may produce interesting insights for intervention in STS. And the same applies to more recent studies on how intervention gets shaped in medical practices.

In his 1997 book *Rationalizing Medical Work*, Marc Berg analyzes the difference between textbook versions and ethnographic accounts of the place and form of interventions in medical decision making. Whereas textbook versions of decision-making practices assume that clinicians first come to a diagnosis that then leads to a decision for a particular clinical intervention in practice, Berg compellingly shows that treatment often begins as a way of tentatively exploring which of the diagnoses that share similar signs or symptoms may be correct. Proposing that diagnosing is a separate phase of decision making and a largely cognitive process is highly similar to assuming that analogical-hypothetical reasoning is the primary style of knowledge production in the sciences (Berg 1997, pp. 20–31). Interestingly, Berg's analysis of medical interventions *as part of* diagnosing resonates with Hacking's analysis of intervening as an important form of knowledge production in the sciences.

Turning such findings reflexively upon the social sciences is important to understand the inappropriateness of Seeley's comparison of social-science interventions that lack a clear diagnosis to social scientists as "a collection of mad doctors." It helps us understand that such interrelating of diagnosing and intervening is *precisely what practicing medicine is often about*, which brings home the point that intervention in the social sciences does not have to be attached to a pre-defined "diagnosis" of what the normative problem is, which is then followed by a social-science intervention. Intervention is reflexively connected to the very production of this diagnosis, or, as Hacking would put it, intervention is about the production of proof about the practice. Drawing on such studies, STS could thus contribute productively to a conceptualization of situated intervention that avoids textbook simplifications. Taking a clinical-*practice* approach to intervention rather than a clinical-*model* approach would help STS to acknowledge, as Edgar Schein put it (1987, p. 29), that "*intervention precedes or is simultaneous with diagnosis*, and that improved diagnosis results from early efforts to intervene." Indeed, the interventions of STS researchers may be better off not being preceded by a sentimental attachment to a grassroots diagnosis of social problems.

Blurring the distinctions between diagnosing and intervening means that the question of relating to the field social scientists study moves away from a dichotomous understanding of power and knowledge that has dominated the debate on social-science interventions for decades. Structuring this debate along this power-knowledge nexus is what Casper Bruun Jensen and Peter Lauritsen (2005, p. 60), following Gilles Deleuze (1991), call a "badly posed problem." They observe two aspects that would qualify the problem as badly posed: it leads to a highly limited range of intellectual positions left for scholars, and this delimits scholarly imagination about the possible relations they could have with their fields. The power-knowledge nexus can be traced back to the work of Marx and Weber and runs through the Becker-Gouldner and public sociology debates and also through some discussions of the normative positioning of STS researchers. It provides infinite degrees but only one kind: though it provides unlimited variations on the *scale* of partisan and objective scholarship, the *relation* between the ends of the scale is always one of less or more of these two extremes.

The alternative figuration of the problem space proposed by STS studies—that of interlocking representing (or diagnosing) and intervening—is largely inspired by feminist studies of science and technology, since feminist STS has done important work in reconfiguring the knowledge-power nexus. Whereas feminism started as a "movement about exclusion—'we need more women in *x*'" (Star 1995, p. 23), thereby reifying rather than problematizing gender categories, with "women in *x*" as "favorite career-building strategies for some" (ibid., p. 24), feminist STS is radically different in that its primary aim is "the ongoing project of unsettling binary oppositions, through philosophical critique and through historical reconstruction of the practices through which particular divisions emerged as foundational to modern technoscientific definitions of the real" (Suchman 2008, p. 140). In relation to the objective knowledge/subjective power binary opposition that paralyzes discussions of the role of sociologists in relation to their fields, one of the most important notions in feminist STS is what Donna Haraway (1991b) calls "situated knowledges." Rather than contrast partiality with objective knowledge, Haraway states that "objectivity turns out to be about particular and specific embodiment, and definitely not about the false vision promising transcendence of all limits and responsibility" (ibid., p. 190). In this sense the notion of objectivity as contradictory to scholarly attachments can be seen as "unlocatable, and so irresponsible" (ibid., p. 191). Being situated, conversely, is needed precisely to accomplish an uncontentious form of objectivity. Or, as Haraway puts it, "the only way to find a larger vision is to be somewhere in particular" (ibid., p. 96).

In this figuration of the problem of the relationship between the social sciences and their fields, the question is not "Whose side are 'we' on?" The question is how located and accountable scholars can create productive partial connections (Strathern 1991) with their fields. The issue is not related to keeping sufficient analytical distance, as again this reduces the matter to a distance scale, leaving nothing but yet another "more/less" answer—"believing in this epistemological chimera closes off many sorts of possible connections" (Jensen and Lauritsen 2005, p. 72). The question is, rather, how scholars can have sufficient connections to a practice they relate to (Latour 1988b) and whether they can "come up with ingenious solutions to the problem of how to become interesting enough for practices to care about" (Jensen and Lauritsen 2005, p. 72).[31] Neither engagement nor objectivity seems to provide the best opportunities for doing so. Rather, the "project of materialized refiguration" (Haraway 1997, p. 23), in which social scientists experiment with different ways of "figuring together, or *configuring*" (Suchman 2008, p. 153) modes of sociological scholarship and the practices studied, may prove fruitful in this regard.

This proposal to pre-empt many of the problems of objectivity and partisanship in discussing the relationship between the social sciences and their fields hardly leads to a set of guidelines or methodology for how to do this research. The point is that scholars learn to "take quite seriously that knowledge is always obtained concretely, and for that matter can never be ensured from the outside, but only through interested interaction" (Jensen and Lauritsen 2005, p. 69). Despite recent attempts to argue the contrary (Barad 2011), such practices of creating material refigurations, as proposed in the work of Haraway, cannot be methodically "followed," because Haraway's "idiosyncratic, hybrid style of speech and writing ... cannot be easily reduced to a package of methodological guidelines" (Prins 1995, p. 362). For these reasons, this approach calls for empirically detailed explorations of new ways of interlocking representing and intervening, for the uncontentious and "agential realism" (Barad 2007) these afford, and for continuous reflexive commitment to the produced situated knowledges and the worlds that scholars generate in intra-action (ibid.) with their fields.

Despite such calls for materialized refiguration, the ways in which STS explores its own implications in world-making is still somewhat limited. I think this is one domain in which STS and social sciences at large still have much to gain from reflexively drawing on the scientific and health care practices studied. STS authors interested in experimenting with refigurations analyze "productive *metaphors*" (Law and Urry 2004, p. 390, emphasis added) that come from complexity theory, plead for "deliberate efforts to structure *inquiry, description, and explanation* to serve social purposes" (Woodhouse et al. 2002, p. 298, emphasis added), "argue for a strategic *dialogue*" (Kember 2003, p. ix, emphasis added) between critics of scientific practices and scientific practitioners, or claim that there is a need to organize "public *debates* on standards" (Callon 2004, p. 131, emphasis added) for the technologies that shape our world. It is striking that many STS scholars restrict themselves to largely *discursive ways* of intervening—with discursive defined in a fairly pre-Foucauldian non-material sense—despite the importance this field has ascribed to other more material modes of intervention in scientific and health care practices (Latour 1988a).

In contrast to these proliferating examples of discursive sociological interventions, the specific approach I develop in this book explores the material reconfiguration of medical practices as a mode of situated intervention. This approach is inspired by the idea that sociological interventions may gain much from getting involved in changing the organization and technologies of medical practice, through which technology can serve as "a crucial, never fully predictable and potentially creative force" (Berg 1998, p. 478). The focus in STS on discursive interventions is surely influenced partly by the kinds of technoscientific practice studied: experimental materialized refigurations may work better in the development of medical information and communications technology than in nuclear energy. Also, I risk enacting another "great divide" here between the material and the discursive,[32] which would be one of the binary oppositions feminist STS would be eager to unsettle. And yet the preference for discursive interventions is not merely asymmetrical with STS sensitivities for the importance of material agency. It often seems to produce a more static notion of normativity that presents "engaged STS" as a resource in such debates. (See, e.g., Fisher 2011.) The turn toward organizational and material explorations of interventionist social-science practices that I put at center stage in this book differs in the sense that such interventions are situated in the normative complexities that are empirically unpacked as well as in the material agency that is part of the refiguration of practice.

Consequently, and in line with the aim of investigating new ways of creating partial connections, this type of research comes with a somewhat unusual set of research practices.

Doing Situated Intervention

The research on situated intervention upon which I draw in this book spans more than ten years. In January of 2001 I joined the Institute of Health, Policy and Management at Erasmus University Rotterdam, pursuing an interest in STS research on (or as) intervention in medical practices. Since then, I have been involved in the development of a hemophilia care center at a large university medical center (2001–2002), in the construction of standardized care pathways in a large hematology/oncology ward at a university hospital (2003–2004), in the development of standardized care pathways for oncology care and elective surgery in a national quality-improvement collaborative that contributed to health care reform aimed at introducing a system of regulated competition (2004–2007), and in the interventionist evaluation of a national collaborative for improving the quality and safety of long-term care (2006–2009). In this period the "methods assemblages" (Law 2004) I worked with ranged widely. In the first three projects, my role was that of a change agent, doing commissioned research, hired to act as project leader for reorganizing care practices. Here the idea was not that an otherwise static practice required transformation, as change is a state that is "already and always in progress" (Blomberg, Suchman, and Trigg 1996, p. 260); it was to articulate and address particular problems in the organization of care. Since such research is not uncommon in the academic institute that employed me, health care organizations and professionals were accustomed to many researchers from this institute carrying out research that was useful to them in one way or another—for example, health economists doing cost-effectiveness studies of clinical trials of innovative treatments. This familiarity of care professionals with the institute and the similarity these actors perceived between my projects and other forms of "useful scholarship" gave the problem of access to medical practices a very specific twist. Although my STS colleagues often had difficulties convincing doctors of the relevance of their obscure ethnographic tendencies,[33] these projects were based on invitations from organizations that viewed this institute as a resource for organizing care practices. In the fourth project, my role was somewhat traditional, as the evaluation of the quality-improvement collaborative addressing long-term care was funded by a research grant by the Netherlands Organization for Health Research and Development (ZonMw). One of the conditions we negotiated was to contribute explicitly to the collaborative: we would run feedback and reflection sessions with those carrying out the improvement projects.

My involvement with developing the hemophilia care center entailed spending about 300 days in the hospital doing ethnographic observations, conducting interviews with nurses, doctors, doctors' assistants, ward managers, pharmacists and patients, having meetings with ICT department staff, care professionals, and care managers, and giving presentations to professionals and patients. Sometimes my observations took me to national meetings of internists-hematologists specialized in hemophilia treatment, to other hemophilia treatment centers in the Netherlands and in the UK, or to international conferences such as the World Federation of Hemophilia Forum. At other times it took me to the ICT department of the hospital or into the homes of patients. The main STS co-researcher on this project was Marc Berg, then the department chair who was directing the research.

Based on the work for the hemophilia care center, the management and medical staff of the hematology/oncology outpatient clinic that the hemophilia care center was part of, asked our department to analyze some persistent problems they faced and to get involved in the needed organizational changes. Though the hemophilia care center is a relatively small unit for one rare disease, the hematology/oncology outpatient clinic and treatment center is a large unit of the university hospital. Annually, approximately 1150 new outpatients come to the clinic about 11,000 times for follow-up consultations. The treatment center administers chemotherapy about 2,100 times and blood transfusions about 2,600 times a year.

Care professionals and patients dealt with many overcrowded outpatient clinics. Clinics ran very late, and at times the treatment center was so jammed that patients had to receive chemotherapy while sitting on a stool, rather than reclining in a chair that can be adjusted to a horizontal position in case the patient reacts badly to the treatment.

In 2003 I started a three-month study of the working problems in the outpatient clinic and treatment center. Combining ethnographic and quantitative approaches, I analyzed the interactions taking place behind the appointments counter, in the consulting room, in the treatment center, in the waiting rooms, and in staff meetings. I carried out 19 days of participant observation; held semi-structured interviews with resident staff, junior doctors, operational management, research nurses, medical secretaries, and medical social workers (23 respondents in all); held focus-group project meetings (twice); gave interactive presentations to nurses (twice), to hematologists (once), to oncologists (once), and to other clinic personnel (twice); and quantified problems by analyzing data from the hospital information system (HIS).

Analyzing HIS data, I could calculate to what extent the clinics were running late, how many patients were scheduled although no regular slot was available (double bookings or over bookings), whether clinics started on time, whether there was an overall balance between the capacity of the clinics and the number of visiting patients, how often doctors canceled clinics, and the variability of these parameters for individual doctors. I also quantified the increase in the number of treatments given at the treatment center in recent years and the distribution of treatment over the various days of the week in the previous three months. I did not look into the rate of "no-shows," as this may be a common problem in wards for less urgent care, but on this ward patients were so ill that they seldom stayed away without notification.

After the first phase of the study, I wrote a proposal for changes that might be made on the ward. When the medical and organizational management approved this analysis and its directions for a solution, over a period of about ten months I spent most of my time on the ward coordinating working groups for hematology and oncology, which were chaired by a professor of hematology and an associate professor of oncology who both served as medical coordinators.[34] These multi-professional groups consisted of the medical coordinators, resident staff members, nurses, doctors' assistants, research nurses, the management of the secretaries, the operational manager of the ward, and me. We met once a week to discuss the progress of the project and to sketch out standardized care trajectories for the large majority of patients. These pathways focused on the interventions that group members proposed to deal with the issues I had identified in the first phase.

In the final two months of the project, I evaluated it by again using a mixed-method design, interviewing professionals and analyzing data from the HIS. (The latter was much less cumbersome the second time, since important parameters were now translated into automatically generated indicators.) In all, I spent about 200 days doing research on the ward in this period. As I mentioned above, Marc Berg was the other main contributor from my department to this project. Substantial contributions also came from Roland Bal, another STS colleague from the institute.

For the third project, I had the dual role of project leader of the national process-redesign project of the quality-improvement collaborative and advisor to one of the large participating teaching hospitals. The national part of the collaborative involved approximately 40 improvement projects in 16 hospitals, and my main work consisted of organizing a series of national conferences for improvement teams, combined with site visits and interviews with project leaders and quality managers (32 in all), which added up to about 180 days of interventionist research. Additionally, I spent about 150 days at the teaching hospital observing care practices, attending meetings of improvement teams, interviewing staff, and attending "project reviews" chaired by the managing and medical directors of the hospital. Initially, Marc Berg was a board member of the national quality-improvement collaborative. Around the halfway point of the study, he was succeeded by Roland Bal.

This study was later extended with a round of follow-up interviews to see how developments in one of the participating hospitals had progressed. I interviewed a specialist nurse, the innovation manager of the hospital, a medical specialist who also chaired one of the specialisms in the hospital, and a division manager. Next, I interviewed a purchaser for the largest insurer in this hospital's catchment area, the development manager, an economic expert at the Dutch Healthcare Authority, and the expert at the Dutch Association of Insurers responsible for developing the purchasing guide for hospital care that insurance companies use.

When evaluating the quality-improvement collaborative for long-term care, I worked with other STS researchers and with quantitative sociologists from the Institute of Health Policy and Management. The latter used surveys to collect outcome data on three levels of the collaborative: the thematic projects in the collaborative, the improvement teams in organizations, and individual clients in those organizations. I carried out participant observations of sixteen working conferences and six meetings of project teams who run the thematic projects in the collaborative, and I interviewed project leaders and health policy makers coordinating the program. With this research design, we intended to analyze the results in terms of effectiveness that the teams seemed to be achieving and, at the same time, to consider what the "results" might be indicating or hiding. I was further involved in meeting with project team leaders and program management in feedback sessions. Because of the more distributed nature of this program, and because I was not involved in changes at the level of health care organizations but rather at the level of the national improvement program, this research was more spread out over time. I must admit that this was a welcome change, allowing for more space to conceptualize work from this and previous projects. Roland Bal was principal investigator for this project; Mathilde Strating and Anna Nieboer were the other main collaborators.

John Law has defined method assemblages as "a combination of reality detector and reality amplifier" (2004, p. 14), and that definition fits the research practices I worked with quite well. Just as it proved problematic to separate diagnosis and intervention in medical work, it was rarely self-evident how findings resulted in interventions, or how interventions produced new knowledge, or even how to separate the two. Intervention turns out to be a highly layered practice that is part and parcel of doing fieldwork, as doing fieldwork in itself begins to interlock representing and intervening. Challenging this dichotomy proved crucial for staying susceptible to opportunities for the initial interlocking of representing and intervening during the period of fieldwork. The co-development of intervention and fieldwork also ensures that situated intervention is not about the implementation of plans, as such implementation would be a problem-ridden route for interventionist researchers, who—like any other actor in the setting—have a limited capacity for carrying out changes according to their wishes (Nickelsen 2009, p. 11). The tension of striving for change while realizing that it will turn out differently than intended cannot be resolved. This makes the role of intervention researchers quite like that of other actors in the field of medicine, and gears this set of method assemblages toward striving for normatively situated interventions—which turn out differently than had been intended.

Structure of the Book

The chapters deal with various experiments with research practices on situated intervention. Though the cases and analyses may seem to progress from empirically detailed practices of the individual actions of patients in a health care setting, moving up to the level of standardization of care trajectories for hospital wards, and further up to market developments and patient-safety programs in national governance arrangements, I do not analyze them as proceeding from a "micro" to a "macro" level. Such ethics of scale would re-introduce the notion that the social has a pre-existing "top" and a pre-existing "bottom" (Latour 1997). I do, however, explore how partial connections have a *history* that is crucial to enabling certain modes of intervention. Although ethnographically inspired STS research does at times have difficulties dealing with the historic depth of sites of knowledge production, "since in general ethnographies deal in very thin time slices" (Bowker 2005, p. 13; also see Engeström 1990), it is precisely this longer time span of analysis and intervention that creates options for different interactions with practices studied.[35] Interventions on the hematology/oncology ward were not possible without the partial connections created on that ward during the project for the hemophilia care center, and my becoming the leader of a national project for developing standardized care trajectories in 16 hospitals would have been unthinkable without my connections to the ward of the university medical center and to some highly esteemed professors of hematology and oncology there. Likewise, the projects were enabled by their connections to my institute. Such associations sometimes interact in quite unforeseen ways; I will return to the history and the interaction of partial connections in the concluding chapter.

In chapter 1, I explore situated intervention in the practice of the hemophilia home treatment carried out under the responsibility of a hemophilia care center. In this case, interventions are strongly connected to STS and sociological research on the issue of compliance and to studies that focus on making work visible. Non-compliance is often conceptualized as a problem in the literature on quality of care, resulting in a plethora of equally unsuccessful compliance enhancement initiatives and cognitive interventions. Medical sociologists and STS researchers question the aim of full compliance, recognizing that patients have to live in many different worlds simultaneously—worlds that at times may challenge their role of patient. By shifting their focus from trying to understand irrational non-compliance to studying achievement of compliance in practice, medical sociologists and STS researchers have opened-up interesting acting space for situating compliance enhancement initiatives in the complexity of patients' life-worlds. In chapter 1, I explore what happens when such insights are translated into material and organizational interventions (for example, by introducing monitoring devices for particularly risky settings) and relate these translations back to the possible gains for sociology and for practices of hemophilia care.

In chapter 2, after discussing the value of experimentally scrutinizing patients' compliance with treatment regimes, I turn to the study of clinicians' compliance with standards. With a rhetorical structure similar to that of the debate about patients' compliance, the low adherence rates of health care professionals to clinical guidelines is often seen by health scientists and policy makers as highly problematic. However, as in the debate on patient adherence, the common "solutions" to improve the success rate of implementation initiatives tend to leave the epistemological status of aggregated medical knowledge untouched. Such initiatives tend to be practically cumbersome, politically desensitized, and conceptually problematic.

They are caught up in a dichotomous understanding of universal clinical knowledge and particular patient characteristics, which is not a productive rendering of the problems encountered in clinical practice. To explore a different notion of standardization, I analyze the experimental interventions in a health-care-improvement project at a hematology/oncology outpatient clinic of the same university hospital. I show that this project articulates the value of situated standardization for both clinical practice and the integrated pathway movement, rather than following the above-mentioned extremes (striving for full rationalization of medical practice and celebrating complexity that boycotts standardization).

In chapter 3, I explore the consequences of situated standardization for the relation between standardization and patient-centeredness. In the literature of medical sociology, "standardization" and "patient-centered care" have been positioned as perfect conceptual opposites. I explore the specificities of this opposition, the limitations of the two concepts, and how a reconceptualization of both concepts could lead to their pragmatic commensurability. Drawing empirically on the development of patient-centered care pathways, I suggest that situated standardization can be helpful for redefining patient-centeredness from a change in professional attitude toward "wholeness," or a procedural focus on patient participation, to a material and organizational characteristic. This proves particularly important because other definitions of patient-centeredness can allow doctors to exert unprecedented power over their patients. If the issues patients, care professionals, and organizations face are put at center stage, care can be made patient-centered in more substantial, contestable, and located ways.

Chapter 4 deals with how sociology can get involved in the enactment of emerging health care markets. Drawing on research on the development of situated standardization through process redesign in a national health-care-quality collaborative, I analyze the possibilities for enacting health care markets as driven by value rather than by cost-saving. Though initially this project was largely successful, I propose that sociological interventions in the construction of markets may be more risky than some scholars suggest. These markets turned out to "work" quite well despite the poor quality of the market devices that I developed to help frame it as value-driven. Later, when the quality of these devices improved, the market focused more on cost-saving. Since many scholars in social studies of markets have argued for the importance of market devices in framing values, it seems important to sensitize the sociological interventions to prevailing *market regimes* and market practices as "forms of the probable" (Thévenot 2002) that are highly consequential for the acting space of social scientists in performing markets.

Sociological interventions in national improvement programs are also the topic of chapter 5, where I focus on a sociological evaluation of a large program devoted to improving the care of older adults. In the evaluation, I initially faced a narrow definition of "useful" research according to which we were supposed to discover the factors that support or hamper the implementation of existing policy agendas. I show how such definitions are unfortunate, since they undo the capacity to complexify the taken-for-granted conceptualizations of the object of study that is crucial for practices of situated intervention. As an alternative to this definition of "usefulness," I explore a focus on multiple ontologies in the making when studying patient safety. Through this focus, social scientists become involved in refiguring the problem space of patient safety, the relations between research subjects and objects, and the existing policy agendas. This role gives social scientists the opportunity to focus on which practices of "effective care" are enacted through different approaches to dealing with patient safety and what their consequences are for the care practices under study. I explore how this focus on multiple ontologies of safety open up new ways for intervention in the quality-improvement collaborative, but also point to the limitations of evaluation as intervention.

In the conclusion I return to the questions raised in this introduction and to the consequences of situated intervention for the normativity of sociological scholarship. I claim that sociologists do not face a normative deficit in the practices they study, but that they have to find new ways of dealing with a normative surfeit, to which they have to relate their own sociological attachments. The strength of situated intervention in elucidating this normative complexity proves fruitful for coming to what I call an *ethics of specificity*. Such an ethics turns a more flexible normativity not into a normative vacuum for sociology, but into a healthy practice of adopting its sociological responses to the practices studied. In this way, sociology not only has more to offer to the practices it studies, but also has more to learn from them.

1   The Stuff of Interventions: Technologies of Compliance in Hemophilia Care

Many older hemophiliacs look back on childhood years of missed opportunities which have resulted in poor quality jobs and long periods of unemployment. The reasons for this are not difficult to find. Effective treatment with concentrated blood products has not been available for long, and children used to be put to bed for weeks of rest after bleeds. ... Nowadays the outlook for even the most severely affected hemophiliac coming up to school age has never been brighter. The child who is intellectually capable of going on to higher education should have as much chance as an unaffected child of doing so.
—Jones 1984, p. 153

Solutions and Their Problems

The quotation above, from one of the founding fathers of modern hemophilia treatment, is typical of popular accounts of how technological developments in medicine affect the lives of patients. As with many other chronic diseases, the story of the development of hemophilia treatment is replete with the rhetoric of progress. In a way, this is not surprising. As in many other cases, the opportunities for patients to participate in activities from which they previously would have been excluded have improved immensely. Also, patients' life expectancies have increased, and while they are alive they will face far fewer problems with joints damaged by "bleeds."

Though advances in medical treatment of chronic diseases seem obvious, seeing them as mere improvements in an otherwise static environment poses its own problems. As authors[1] from the field of STS have observed when researching the development of medical treatment, new forms of care or the introduction of new devices often engender new issues in the sociotechnical interplay of patients, doctors, devices, and institutions.

Analyzing new forms of treatment and their consequences has been a main aim for scientific fields like medical sociology and, more recently, STS.

This analytical work has led to detailed studies of the complexities such developments entail for patients and care providers. It has at times also led to criticism of existing care practices and to suggestions for addressing the problems analyzed. However, it has less often resulted in STS researchers' becoming directly involved in the design and development of care practices.

In this chapter I investigate some of the issues that arise when intervening in the proactive construction of a specific form of hemophilia care. I explore how hemophilia care can be productively reconfigured through entangling it with STS insights, and how such entanglements have consequences for debates on compliance and normativity in STS. I begin by turning to the question of *how* situated intervention may come about in practice by analyzing my involvements in the development of a hemophilia care center.

Reconfigured Care, Different Patients, Changed Doctors: Toward Home Treatment of Hemophilia

Hemophilia is a disorder that makes a patient bleed either spontaneously or after intense activity. "Bleeds" occur as a result of a deficiency of coagulation factors in the blood that are responsible for blood clotting. With the development of pharmaceutical substitutes for coagulation factors, the duration of bleed treatment has decreased from several days or weeks of hospitalization to almost immediate results following an injection of medication. This has cleared the way for one of the most remarkable events in the history of hemophilia treatment: the change from hospital treatment to home treatment.[2]

Until the 1960s, hemophilia patients had to be treated in hospitals, having their joints immobilized and receiving blood transfusions to allow the bleeding to subside or, from 1966 on, receiving concentrated blood products such as cryoprecipitate.[3] Now they can take a training course that teaches them how to self-diagnose bleeds and administer coagulation factor concentrates at home, either ad hoc or as prophylactic treatment.[4] Since virtually every severe hemophiliac undergoes this training, for the vast majority of bleeds patients are treated *under the supervision of* a hemophilia care center.

With the transfer of hemophilia treatment from the hospital to the home (or to the workplace, or to a vacation setting), medical professionals had to adjust to their new role of long-distance controllers of care. They witnessed a substantial discrepancy between recommended treatment and patients' actual practice in home treatment, and were concerned about patients' compliance with or adherence to treatment advice.[5]

I became involved in this issue when care providers from a hemophilia care center approached the research group I belonged to.[6] The physicians were facing a major policy change, intended to restructure the organization of hemophilia care in the Netherlands. They wanted to "hire us in" to help them make the changes needed to meet the new policy requirements. A few years earlier, the Minister of Health had asked hemophilia doctors to indicate what was crucial for ensuring high-quality treatment. The doctors suggested the following: a multidisciplinary care team, guaranteed specialized care 24 hours a day, regular consults with patients (at least once a year), and plans per individual patient indicating preferred treatment per type of injury. The minister noted these requirements and fixed them as the new treatment norm (Borst-Eilers 1999). This presented hemophilia doctors with a substantial problem, as the new policy was based on their dreams of the organization of care in an ideal world rather than on actual work practices. At one of the first meetings, Peter Linden, the internist-hematologist who was my main contact in the project, told me that his foremost concern was not with meeting the newly imposed criteria but rather with the situation of home treatment. As he put it, "nobody knows what's actually going on there."

Care providers, still responsible for the treatment now shifted to the home setting, expressed serious concern for the risks that follow undertreatment, including long-term joint damage and potential death of the patient. With the change to home treatment, health care professionals had done their best to make the patients feel responsible for their own treatment, but effectively and legally they still carried the responsibility as deliverers of care. Dr. Linden told me the tragic story of a patient who was brought into the hospital in a critical state. Mounting his bicycle to leave for work, the patient had bumped his head on the garden shed. He had gone back inside his home and had given himself only about a third of the amount of coagulation factor concentrates prescribed in his treatment plan for a head bleed. At work, he became unwell. By the time he was brought to the hospital, it was too late to save his life. The hematologist also used this example of a highly preventable, clumsy death to show his medical students that accidents *can* happen—with drastic consequences—and to emphasize the weighty task they would face in enhancing compliance.[7]

Besides the obvious problems of under-treatment, doctors and nurses similarly feared the risks of over-treatment, since they were constantly maneuvering within a scarcity of medication and funds.[8] Blood-derived medication depends on the availability of donor blood, of which there is a general shortage.[9] Although the introduction in 1993 of "copy-DNA" or recombinant coagulation factor concentrates was expected to provide a potentially unlimited supply of safe medication, this promise was initially not redeemed, and was followed by periods of serious worldwide shortage well into the new millennium (Traore et al. 2014). Recombinant coagulation factor concentrates are not made from human blood, but through DNA manipulation of hamster cells. This reduces the risk of all kinds of infections and supply problems that may arise when using human products. Quite regularly, however, pharmaceutical companies announced problems in the production process with the result that their products became unavailable for several months. Though blood-derived medication with the same effect was generally available, it was risky to make patients switch between products. A patient might develop an inhibitor to all coagulation factors, which makes treatment largely ineffective, and for a young patient who had used only recombinant medication switching to blood products meant being exposed for the first time to all the associated infection risks.[10] Therefore, doctors and nurses had to take strong action in case of supply problems to distribute recombinant products to children, and only older patients could have their medication changed back to blood-derived clotting factor.

Even now that the production of recombinant coagulation factor concentrates has become more stable, and the availability of products is no longer a major concern in Western health care settings, care providers (and patients) are still sensitive to the financial aspects of extremely expensive medication. On various occasions in the project, providers (and patients) emphasized the exorbitant costs of treatment: tens of thousands of euros per patient per year. Both doctors and patients compared the treatment to "shooting up a Mercedes a year." Though compliance and limiting over-consumption had been matters of concern for quite some time, they became more important as a result of the above-mentioned substantial changes in the policy demands that were imposed on the hemophilia care centers by the Ministry of Health. The problem space of quality improvement in hemophilia care seemed to be framed in classical biomedical terms, with the fact that patients do not follow medical orders as prescribed in treatment plans a main issue. I realized early on in the project that this problem space would not allow for any action repertoires other than ensuring that patients would follow treatment, which was not quite the kind of solution I could easily relate to. Still, how this problem space should be refigured was left to be found out in the quality-improvement experiment.

Dealing with Non-Compliance

Non-compliance is mainly seen as a *problem per se* in literature on the treatment of chronic diseases. In *Tools of Care*, Dick Willems states that this has resulted in the situation in which "compliance enhancement has become a basic principle of good medical practice" (1995, p. 126). The prevalence of compliance-enhancement initiatives, however, is hardly any guarantee of success. As meta-reviews of randomized controlled trials (RCTs) of enhancement interventions continue to show, low adherence to prescribed treatments is "ubiquitous." McDonald, Garg, and Haynes (2002, p. 2868) conclude that "the full benefit of medications cannot be realized at currently achievable levels of adherence; therefore, more studies of innovative approaches to assist patients to follow prescriptions for medications are needed." It is somewhat ironic that this conclusion follows an extensive literature search showing that "even the most effective interventions [to enhance compliance] had modest effects" (ibid.). Thus, even though striving for full compliance as an optimal state of treatment has proved extremely problematic,[11] it is still regarded as the dominant assumption in the medical literature on adherence, with more enhancement tools and maximum compliance the undisputed goals. This assumption is important for the dominant repertoire on non-compliance that I will call the *repertoire of distrust*.

The Repertoire of Distrust
In the medical literature, non-compliance is often analyzed in terms of the "underlying cognitive mechanisms" causing the "problem." "Patients *forget* their medication. Perhaps they have an unspoken *resistance* against it and *think the disease is over* as soon as their symptoms disappear."[12] (Willems 2001, p. 64) Accordingly, attempts to enhance compliance are often expressed in terminology that produces an "atmosphere of unmasking, of distrust and of authority" (Willems 1995, p. 127). These cognitive explanations result in strategies of improvement for patients' knowledge of their disease, and for improving their attitude by providing better information on treatment. Information flyers are not the only resource of this repertoire. In the treatment of chronic diseases, treatments plans, medication journals, examinations, diplomas, and the signing of contracts by patients and care providers are common interventions focused on improving patients' knowledge of their disease and overcoming cognitive hindrances to full compliance. An interesting feature of this repertoire is that it focuses on *treatment as planned*—that is, treatment as defined in treatment plans, at a

considerable distance from the practices of care delivery. It is this distance in the repertoire of distrust that seems to produce *evidence-based failures* for dealing with the issue of compliance. Because I was familiar with sociological critiques of this repertoire of distrust and of the notion of compliance (Lutfey 2005; Lutfey and Wishner 1999; Conrad 1985, 1987), I took the low success rates of these compliance-enhancement initiatives as a starting point for reflecting on the *causes* of the poor track record. To do so I turned to *home treatment as embodied practice.*

Events in Hemophilia Home Treatment

In the hemophilia-care-center project, there was no need to introduce this empirical turn to practices of home treatment, as I do in this chapter. The health care professionals strongly encouraged me to study patients at home. They had experienced that even when a patient and a care provider carefully negotiated an annual treatment plan that made sense to both parties, in practice treatment actions deviated substantially from the negotiated plan. Because the care providers were eager to have me first quantify this "substantial deviation," I called in a colleague from my institute[13] who analyzed the data that patients had entered in their home treatment journals and the hemophilia nurse had entered into a database. Interestingly, though treatment data had been collected rigorously for years, the data had not been analyzed before. We focused on sixteen severe patients, with less than 1 percent active coagulation factor in their blood, as they would have largely similar treatment plans. We analyzed their treatment in 4,573 events registered for the sixteen patients over a five-year period. We analyzed the data per type of bleed (e.g., ankle bleeds) and specified both the number of times medication was administered and the average dose of medication for the entire episode. We also analyzed the treatment patterns per patient. All data showed substantial variation. (See figure 1.1.) Patients with similar treatment plans and types of bleeds treated themselves very differently. Whereas some patients always treated their bleeds with the same dose of coagulation factor concentrates, others varied widely in the treatment they administered.

I discussed these outcomes with the care professionals involved. Because they knew all the patients well, they could explain quite a few variations arising from working situations, sports activities, and other factors. However, there were quite a few differences that were not easily explained. Care professionals were thus very interested in finding out what was happening with treatment in patients' homes.

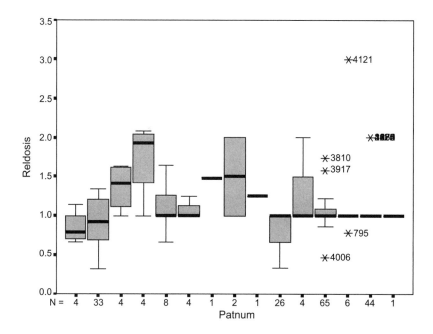

Figure 1.1
Box plot averages of relative dose (reldosis) coagulation factor concentrates per elbow bleed per patient (patnum).

This curiosity was fanned by the fact that hemophilia treatment professionals hold a somewhat unusual position. Whereas chronic patients are a constant group, highly experienced in dealing with their disease, hemophilia doctors often change on the scene. Because of hemophilia's low incidence, hemophilia treatment is concentrated in university medical centers, even though scientifically the development of treatment methods is rather unexciting. For doctors there is not much to gain in terms of academic career development by specializing in hemophilia care. Although some truly committed care professionals have chosen this patient category despite opportunities in more scientifically rewarding diseases, the organization of specialized hemophilia care training in university hospitals also contributes to the fairly high turnover of care providers, in further contrast to the more stable and central position of patients. This strong position for patients was enacted even more firmly by an influential patient alliance, the Dutch Association of Hemophilia Patients. With a membership rate of about 95 percent of Dutch hemophilia patients, they could act (and were seen) as a very powerful agent. Showing that the othering of expertise is

not done only by biomedically focused doctors, one patient noted the position of one of the newer care providers in the center: "This doctor has just
recently joined us." Here Howard Becker's sensitivity to the "hierarchy of
credibility" (1967) seemed unexpectedly relevant to how patients sometimes ranked medical expertise and authority far lower than their own,
based on the high turnover of specialists. This situation also seemed a good
moment to be reminded of Becker's warning to avoid sociological sentimentality (ibid.) in a sociological research practice that is inclined to study
the marginalized position of *patients*. Given the marginalization of *professionals* in this somewhat unusual care setting, both health care professionals and I felt that studying the practice of home treatment might become
part of a welcome experiment that could perhaps help professionals to alter
this balance slightly.

Following a path proposed by various STS authors (Thévenot 1993;
Willems 2000; Conein et al. 1993), I decided to focus the analysis of present practices of home treatment on the ways in which humans and non-
humans share the coordination work needed to bring about a particular
practice of home treatment. I also followed the call for symmetry by studying events in both compliance and non-compliance as phenomena needing further analysis (Willems 2001).

Situated (Ir)rationalities

If you want to get a piercing done, and you want it to work out well, you have to
take a considerable booster shot of clotting factors. I think that's going too far;
shooting up €500 just for a piercing.
—Marco van Veen, interviewed patient[14]

One of the internists I met during the project came from the largest hemophilia care center in the Netherlands. He was rather cynical about the competence of patients to treat themselves. "Patients just do whatever they feel
like," he said while talking about home treatment. This statement turned
out to be widely off the mark during the observations and interviews of
patients at home. One of the first things that became apparent was that
those who suffer from a chronic illness spend a relatively short period of
time in the role of patient (Conrad 1985, 1987). They have to combine a
variety of "worlds" in which they play various—not necessarily complementary—roles. It was obvious that the homes and other personal settings
of hemophilia patients were quite different from the previous locus of treatment: a university hospital. This insight was, of course, nothing new, and

care providers recognized that such was the case when home treatment began. It was therefore embedded in the above-mentioned training program, in the exam patients had to pass, and in the patient's signed contract. The embedding of this insight served the aims of facilitating "correct" treatment at home and ensuring a clear distribution of liability. In an interview, one patient said:

Before I started home treatment I had some training in injections. They checked if I was doing everything right. It was mainly practical. When you treat yourself at home, you mustn't panic. The chance of reactions [to medication] was bigger at the time, but that didn't bother me much. Still, it was a risk you took home. So you have to be sure you can deal with it. What I remember most were the practical things: put stuff down neatly and make sure your hands are clean. And of course, the training is also there to limit the doctor's liability as much as possible, because if things go wrong then the doctor could say: "Look, it's not our fault, because we told you this hundreds of times."

Various interventions in the establishment of home treatment were mainly geared to distributing formal legal responsibilities or informing and educating patients about their treatment. There is, however, a problem with the temporality and spatiality of these interventions: though introduced in a particular time and in a particular place, they take effect later and in a different location. It is this disparity in time and space and the absence of (a connection to) the intervention in the actual event of treatment that often renders it useless. The absence of a material connection between the actual events of treatment to these initiatives deprives them of their potential to coordinate the various roles hemophilia patients are playing.

In the repertoire of distrust, the medically situated views of (ir)rationality and of its concurrent disciplining tendencies suppose that unknowledgeable patients are unable to be like fully compliant "model patients" and thus ignorantly harm themselves. We found that patients are aware of the existence of "model patients," but that their deviations from the ideal are often far from arbitrary and do not result from incompetence or cognitively destructive tendencies. For example, one patient said:

I run my own business, so my time is valuable. And since my health is relatively good, I don't like unnecessary exams. I want to have a few useful things examined, but not for the sake of research. I've made good agreements with Dr. Linden about it. So, as far as that goes, I might not be their model patient. I'm calm, so in that sense maybe I am, but they would most like to see everyone every six months for all kinds of nice analyses. I've set that to once a year. Good enough for me, because I told them I'd always come by if something went wrong. Every year I hear the same thing at my checkup. I need them for the stuff [medication], and as backup in case something goes wrong.

The "model" to which patients should adhere encounters strong competition from other roles played in other worlds in the patient's life that enact different expectations.[15] These other roles may seriously test the "alliance" between care center and patient that is needed for a patient to live the role of hemophiliac. In the interviews, several patients mentioned situations in which they perceived the demands of others as opposing the demands of treatment—for example, taking part in gym class at school, or taking part in a decathlon organized by a patient's neighbors. However, the alliance also, at times, received unexpected support where it could have been fractured. Here is an example:

A few weeks ago, at school, we had to lug a bunch of tables from the first floor downstairs for an exam. I wanted to help carry, I thought it wouldn't be a problem, but a few colleagues said, "Why don't you do the corridor, and we'll do the stairs." Then I thought, okay, they've got a point there.

In this case the role of collegial school teacher conflicts with the role of hemophiliac, and the school setting together with the obvious urgency of getting things ready for an exam challenges the durability of the alliance between the patient and the care center. It has been noted that "improving the success of a treatment programme not only demands strengthening the alliance between patient and programme, but also between the programme and the patient's relatives and other significant persons" (Willems 1995, p. 135). In this case the colleagues can help coordinate the roles and worlds that have to be brought together.

Delegating the construction of alliances to humans may be a fruitful approach in some respects, but failing to including non-humans may limit the durability of the alliance between patient and care center. Similarly, defining non-adherence as a "cognitive problem" ignores the way coordination can be obstructed by *materialities*, as in the following excerpt from an interview:

I was still working in an office then. I would take factor VIII that I kept in the fridge there, with my name on the bottle. If I had a bleed, I'd stay inside. They'd reserved a room for me for this. It saved time.

For treatment to be carried out safely, it was important that a second person was present to intervene in case of an allergic reaction to medication. This need conflicts with the specificities of the workplace: the desire for privacy and the corporate ideal of labor productivity are afforded at the expense of the safety of hemophilia care.

Symmetrically studying the mysteries of both non-compliance *and* compliance proved fruitful for gaining an understanding of the complexity of the worlds patients have to coordinate in the practice of hemophilia home treatment. These insights were valuable when experimenting with interventions to change these practices. Experimental interventions cannot aim at uncritically or imprecisely enhancing adherence, but should explicitly contribute to *coordinating the various worlds patients inhabit in those instances where it seems to matter most.* The experiments consisted of a range of developments, including designing a digital version of the logbook of medication administered at home and an online portal for communication between patients and care centers. Here, I focus on two modest yet interesting interventions: the introduction of a small but powerful temperature-monitoring device and the development of a multidisciplinary hemophilia consulting hour.

Experiments in the Practice of Hemophilia Care

As we observed during the home treatment study, vacations pose by far the biggest challenges for coordinating the various worlds patients inhabit. The arrival of coagulation factor concentrates has enabled patients to bring medication along to their vacation destination and carry on treatment somewhere even more remote from the hospital than the usual home setting. Despite this substantial relocation of care, patients are expected to treat themselves on vacation much as they would do at home—or rather, as they would in hospital. On top of that, they are supposed to ensure suitable conditions for transporting and storing their medication on their stay. These conditions are fairly demanding: to remain efficacious, coagulation factor concentrates must be kept in a cool place, preferably a vibration-free industrial refrigerator. With the displacement of care to the vacation setting, the norms of professional cooling equipment, the careful chain of transport by pharmaceutical companies before the medication arrives in the center,[16] and all the safety regulations that a hospital pharmacy has to adhere to are substituted for by a portable cool box or a small daypack equipped with a cooling compartment and removable cooling elements. This barely coordinates the worlds of the hemophiliac and the vacationer, and sometimes it leads to serious treatment problems. One patient, Mr. Hilhorst, explained:

I had an ankle bleed over there that lasted almost a week. In that week I took a lot of medication. Four weeks in four different campsites and all that time I was sitting in the same chair. I shot up 2,000 units every day, but it wouldn't stop. We looked for a local treatment center after a day or two, but then it started improving slowly. Probably the drug didn't work. Perhaps it was too warm. We kept it in a bag with cooling elements, but it was over 30°C outside. I think that we should have swapped [the cooling elements] every day, and I must have forgotten. I've been sloppy with that.

interviewer: Did you check afterwards if the temperature was the actual problem?
Mr. Hilhorst: No, I didn't check.

The setting of beaches, campsites, high temperatures, cooling elements and relaxed vacationers provided strong challenges to the effectiveness of this event of hemophilia care.

Similarly challenging treatment events were analyzed to further specify who found the "problems" actually "problematic." Of course, one could argue that this state of affairs is problematic only for hemophilia doctors, and that it looks like a dream come true for sociologists of deviance propagating the notion that noncompliance with treatment, "supports people's desire for independence and autonomy" (Conrad 1987, p. 15) in contrast to focusing on compliance—a notion that is merely "conceived to solve the doctor's problem" (ibid.). In view of the long history of seeing non-compliance with treatment as deviance to be corrected, it is easy to understand scholarly distrust of compliance-enhancement initiatives. When such a sentiment turns into sentimentality, any compliance-enhancing intervention would be an illegitimate, unfair challenge to patients' autonomy. Though this scholarly position may sound an unlikely caricature of sociological attachments, this is precisely the criticism I received on presenting this situation at an STS forum. The question raised was "But aren't you just disciplining the patients?!" In terms similar to the risks Robert Straus pointed out in 1957 for doing sociology *in* medicine, I was accused of becoming an insider in the medical profession, talking, acting, and thinking like a doctor. That charge was strengthened by the fact that I did not refrain from using the highly dubious notion of "compliance" rather than its more accepted sociological counterpart, "adherence." As the sociologist Karen Lutfey and the clinician William Wishner argue (1999, p. 635), "the term 'compliance' suggests a restricted medical-centered model of behavior, while the alternative 'adherence' implies that patients have more autonomy in defining and following their medical treatments." I tend to be sympathetic to this sociological attachment, even when taking the extreme position that autonomous patients should be free to prefer death over a medicalized life—the ultimate risk of treatment with ineffective medication. I am inspired by sociological work that calls notions of treatment or even health into question as cultural images that are "at once wholly mainstream and impossible to attain" (Metzl 2010, p. 2). Yet such freedom to be what Jonathan Metzl and Anna Kirkland (2010) call "against health" may also have implications for the risks other patients face during treatment. In Mr. Hilhorst's case, he only used a great deal of scarce and costly factor VIII; he also exposed the medication to high temperatures and did not actually check whether it had lost its efficacy. According to Dutch pharmacy law, clotting agents brought back unused from vacation trips must be discarded. Once drugs have left the controlled setting of professional care, administering them to other patients is considered too risky. Yet, because the high cost and scarcity of clotting factors, this is exactly what all hemophilia care centers did. Although they consider it too risky to hand out this medication for home treatment, care professionals in hospitals do administer the drugs for emergency bleeds or as prophylaxis for surgery. Though such events are clinically more dangerous, administering medication that has been taken back from patients is considered safer in the highly controlled and monitored setting of the clinic. In such arrangements, articulating the "autonomy" of vacationing patients actually jeopardizes the effectiveness of the treatment of other patients. On these grounds, it seemed a good situation for an experimental intervention that would enact the world and the responsibilities of the hemophiliac more strongly, thereby enhancing compliance with the way medication is supposed to be handled. Without strongly articulating the world of the hemophiliac, the world of the vacation traveler would prevail to such an extent that it would jeopardize medication safety dramatically.

Peter Linden, the internist-hematologist heading the project, directed my attention to a device that might play an important coordinating role: TechTemp loggers, devices that register temperatures at regular intervals (figure 1.2). We began an experiment to see if loggers could induce proper handling of medication. We added a logger to sealed packages of patients' medication. We informed the patients that a temperature logger was in their travel pack, and that if they returned unused medication we would check the temperatures that their drugs had been exposed to. I wrote a small research protocol for the pilot that included the rule that every time one of our two loggers became re-available, it would be given to the first patient coming in for a travel pack.

The experiment had two interesting results. First, in several instances the returned medication had been exposed to temperatures that, according to the instructions for use, were not acceptable. This surprised the nurse, who had been unhappy about having to hand out loggers to patients she felt were "reliable." Her expectations were influenced by ethnicity and vacation destination: she expected a middle-aged Dutch man going to France on a short break would face less risk than a man of Moroccan origin driving to

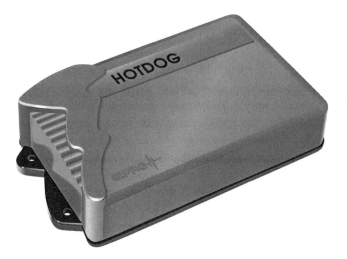

Figure 1.2
TechTemp temperature logger. Courtesy of Elpro.

his homeland for a six-week summer vacation. Since she thought every-thing would go well, she feared that the experiment would fail because the loggers would not produce any interesting data. I was unable to assess the appropriateness of her expectations, but it turned out that patients she con-sidered reliable were at least also exposing their medication to high tem-peratures. Second, the loggers, though intended only to log temperature, proved to be agential in altering the way patients handled medication. On his first vacation trip, a particularly "reliable" patient surprised both the nurse and himself by exposing his medication to excessively high tempera-tures. He received a logger again when he came in for another travel pack a few months later. After his second trip, he was quite sure that nothing had gone wrong with the medication, but his second pack too had to be thrown out because the medication had been exposed to temperatures that were *too low*—at one point, below 0°C. The patient had kept the medication in his ski box on top of his car while en route to his skiing destination, and also at night. Though the result for the medication was the same—both batches had gone to waste—this event demonstrates that the logger can be a power-ful actor. Including it is consequential in the remote landscape of a vacation setting. By registering temperatures, it facilitated coordination between the world of strict safety regulations and the world of relaxing vacations. Even when medication was exposed to overly high or low temperatures, this no longer jeopardized the effective treatment of other patients, nor did it lead to discarding unacceptable amounts of usable medication. The logger thereby confined the risk of inappropriate handling of medication by the autonomous individual patient.

Though adding the logger to the vacation event influenced the actions of this patient to some extent, it did not prevent the medication from getting discarded. This sparked a discussion of whether the world of the hemophilia patient could be enacted more strongly if we developed a logger that not only registers temperature but also acts as an alarm, on behalf of the care center—for example by beeping—to warn patients when they are exposing their medication to excessively high or low temperatures. This could prevent the waste of scarce and expensive medication. At present it is unresolved whether such an extended coordination mechanism would be too much of a disciplinary encroachment on the patient's vacation, or if it could be justified by the risk of treating future patients with ineffective medication. It seems that this setting could warrant a stronger intervention, but it would require further discussions among patients, care professionals, and policy actors.

Some tensions that may emerge from this experimental intervention are that, in order to provide functionalities like alarms we would have to look for other loggers that can do this already, or get involved in redesigning our current loggers, which would provide all kinds of other constraints of intervention and design. Additionally, although the new logger might be a lifesaver, it might also lead to shifting both responsibility and cost completely to hemophilia patients.[17] If the costs of wasted medication could be claimed from patients, this could be seen as a strong incentive for enhancing compliance, but we would have to analyze such shifts in responsibility in the light of strong enactments of self-reliance for hemophilia patients. For example, young patients are taught self-confidence at "survival camps." These camps are sponsored by pharmaceutical companies, which are, of course, strongly interested in enacting patients as "self-reliant" and "certain," especially when these "selves" depend on the pharmaceutically intensive practice of prophylactic home treatment. Similar shifts in responsibility and discipline, combined with a previously unthinkable availability of products, have been analyzed in relation to the "epidemic" of obesity in the United States. It has been noted that "the neoliberal shift in personhood from citizen to consumer encourages (over)eating at the same time that neoliberal notions of discipline vilify it" and that "those who can achieve thinness amidst this plenty are imbued with the rationality and self-discipline of perfect subjects, who in some sense contribute to the more generalized sense of deservingness that characterizes US culture today" (Guthman and DuPuis 2006, p. 427).

I had similar concerns about the survival camps that rendered hemophiliacs self-reliant but perhaps also impossibly responsible and dependent. Yet the pediatrician from the care center, while discussing the counterintuitive practice of young people with bleeding disorders doing hazardous things such as abseiling (rappelling down a rock face) and the ironies of enacting self-reliance that perfectly matched pharmaceutical dependence and maximum use of medication, made it clear to me that she saw no reason for conflict. Rather, she stated, it was an important moment for these young individuals to break out of the overprotective atmosphere that their parents often created for them. I was clearly unable to "intervene" here, since I could not convince anyone that such camps may at least be problematic in some ways.

The experiment with temperature loggers shows that intervening in the coordination of care can produce both new knowledge and new scholarly attachments in relation to the notion of compliance, as well as indicate the limits to calling into question others' prevailing attachments. Instead of focusing on the problems of restricting patient autonomy, the experiment allows for further specifying what issues may warrant compliance-enhancement initiatives and what issues are better left to patients to maneuver. This experiment therefore indicates that exploring the possible role of small technologies in coordinating complexity in home treatment practices can lead to interesting new social-science understandings and interventions. It also shows that certain issues that social scientists would like to open up for debate, such as the normative and financial high costs of a sentimental attachment to enacting patients' self-reliance, can easily remain closed off, making the interventions always tricky and unpredictable and with their own possible risks of—in this case—shifting the burden of wasted medication to patients.

But such experiments are not limited to small technological devices. The role of the hemophilia nurse seemed exceptionally important during my analysis of work at the hemophilia care center, but this nursing work was largely invisible and could benefit from further articulation. During my observations, I noticed numerous continuous small interferences in treatment during the interactions between hemophilia nurses and patients coming in to collect their medication. Handing out medication could be seen as a routine that any qualified pharmacy employee could carry out. And it wasn't only ward management that saw it that way; one of the quotations above also indicates that patients saw nurses as merely handing out their "stuff." Yet hemophilia nurses insisted on doing this "unfit" work, to the great dissatisfaction of nursing management and other nurses on the ward, who qualified the conversations arising in this setting as merely "chatting with patients." During these apparently casual exchanges, hemophilia nurses often found out clinically relevant information and could give treatment advice accordingly. If a nurse asked a patient how he was doing, and the patient said that he was feeling stressed about exams, the nurse knew that stress was an indicator of a higher risk of bleeds, and that a slight increase in the dose of prophylactic treatment could be beneficial. Sensitized to the importance of articulating and accommodating "invisible work" by the work of Lucy Suchman (2000, 1995) and of Susan Leigh Star and Anselm Strauss (1999), I realized that this work could probably gain legitimacy by providing a formal space for such encounters.

That insight contributed to the installation of a multidisciplinary hemophilia clinic, including one nurse-led clinic and one for the physiotherapist. This clinic is an example of an intervention that seemed substantially important to coordinating and negotiating the worlds of hemophilia patients and other roles. The aim of the consulting hour was not merely to inform or "educate" patients, but to formalize the role of the hemophilia nurse in communicating with patients to spot emerging difficulties. Furthermore, scheduling this clinic parallel to the hematologist's surgery hours intensified cooperation between patients and nurses and cooperation between nurses and hematologists. In this experiment, the threat to the legitimacy of nurses taking substantial non-standardized action in guiding patients did not come from clinicians defending their professional autonomy. Doctors, especially those in training, were used to hemophilia nurses correcting their prescribed treatment since the nurses simply had far more expertise in these matters. Rather, the threat came, perhaps unexpectedly, from colleagues who saw the hemophilia nurses as too independent and insufficiently integrated in the totality of the ward (Zuiderent 2002). "We shouldn't return to the situation where hemophilia is something completely different, with different privileges and all," the head nurse of the hematology/oncology outpatient clinic and treatment center told me. "That was the case when I came here," she noted, "and I was told that was exactly the problem with this clinic!" She went on to say that, at the time, "hemophilia nurse" was not a registered profession in the Netherlands, and the nurse doing this work was included as much as possible in job rotations to the other positions in the clinic. So although the installation of the hemophilia clinic may seem a minimal intervention, it had consequences for legitimizing crucial hemophilia nursing work on the ward.

A final advantage of installing the hemophilia surgery hour was that patients who had been seen by various doctors during surgery hours that were spread out over the week, would meet again, at least while waiting for the consult with the hematologist, the physiotherapist, or the hemophilia nurse. In the days of hospital treatment, patients also brought issues to the hospital that were relevant to how they lived with their disease. This not only hospitalized the patients but also socialized the hospital, as part of "'smuggling' patient perspectives and competences into the daily work of the physician" (Willems 2000, p. 29). Bringing patients and health care professionals back into more structured contact might help to reduce the increased distance[18] that had arisen between the care center and its patients as a result of the development of home treatment. Reducing this distance may facilitate the shift from mere compliance enhancement to finding ways to coordinate the complex worlds that may collide in treatment practice.

Addressing this topic in a talk given to patients and health care professionals at the official opening of the hemophilia care center, I tried to explain the aim of making the clinic more than just a place to discuss "issues of non-compliance." Quoting from their interviews and affirming that people with hemophilia simply cannot be expected to be "model patients," I presented the consultancy hour as an opportunity to discuss the complexity patients face during home treatment. This indicates that conceptualizing "hired in" research practices as the "willingness on the part of social researchers to allow their work to be assessed and evaluated in the theoretical terms current in the field" (Downey and Lucena 1997, p. 119) may imply an overly unidirectional consequence for STS researchers that is not necessarily encountered. To distinguish research on situated intervention from sociology that works in pre-set problem spaces or organizational consultancy, I would claim, there should be a *mutual willingness* and interest of various parties to be inspired and "contaminated" by one another's practices. On this note, let me return to some of the consequences of these experiments for conceptualizing situated intervention and normativity in sociological research.

Unsentimental Social Science and Situated Compliance Enhancement

The interaction between scholars working on the terms of actors in a field they only partly belong to has been classified as the problem of the "outsider within." Though this notion was initially developed to analyze the specifics of the outsider within the *discipline of sociology* (Collins 1986), its importance has mainly been ascribed to the more general implications for the relation between sociologists and their fields. As Patricia Hill Collins wrote (1986, p. S29):

[T]he creative tension of outsider within status ... is one where intellectuals learn to trust their own personal and cultural biographies as significant sources of knowledge. In contrast to approaches that require submerging these dimensions of self in the process of becoming an allegedly unbiased, objective social scientist, outsiders within bring these ways of knowing back into the research process.

This focus on this more general point, generally defined as the ability to wear "the double glasses of insider and outsider" (Star 1995, p. 1), has largely been productive, but it has also led to the loss of some aspects of Collins's conceptualization specific to the potentiality of being an African-American feminist sociologist in an at times traditionally oriented field. Where, as Collins puts it, this notion was initially an "apt description of individuals like myself who found ourselves caught between groups of unequal power" (1999, p. 85), it has become more of a "personal identity category ... [of which the] logical conclusion means that everyone can now claim 'outsider within' identity" (ibid., p. 86). This looser notion of the outsider within, unconnected to power relations between groups, has produced two problems. First, as Collins points out (ibid., pp. 87–88), "people who claim 'outsider within' identities can become hot commodities in social institutions that want the illusion of difference without the difficult effort needed to change actual power relations." To avoid such a simplified notion of difference and inclusion, Collins emphasizes the importance of maintaining the collective nature of an outsider-within position. The second related problem is that this notion may be highly productive in settings where clearly identified unequal power relations exist between groups but may at other times be more problematic. In more ambiguous settings, it runs the risk of reifying both outside and inside categories, thereby possibly reducing the options for interesting reconfigurations of attachments for the various actors involved.

In the case of experimental interventions in the practice of hemophilia care, these experiments were inspired by sociological research into the problems of compliance, issues related to the coordination of worlds patients live in, and studies on making work visible. They were, however, equally informed by the risky experiences of both care professionals and noncompliant patients, which, in turn, seemed to problematize sociological critiques of compliance enhancement. Instead of positioning myself as a sociological outsider problematizing compliance in the world of clinical insiders aiming for compliance, situated intervention afforded the production of different compliance-enhancement practices. Consequently, compliance enhancement was done very differently in the case of risky medication-handling in a vacation setting than when dealing with the tensions of following treatment plans in the complexity of a workplace or family setting. Considering the difficulties people face in combining their "being a patient" with the other roles they play, full compliance *and* full autonomy become equally unattainable and undesirable. This is exactly what made the experiments that dealt with a particular (and particularly problematic) issue in hemophilia home treatment interesting to me and to health care professionals and patients. Assessing interventions on the basis of their contribution to the coordination of the worlds patients inhabit and indicating the instances where stronger compliance enhancement may be worth pursuing proved interesting for problematizing a conceptualization of compliance as something medical practices should have "more" or "less" of. Seeing experimental interventions as attempts to deal with the "outsider-within" question would make it harder to move away from the more/less compliance debate and limit the scholarly imagination to experiment with a less dichotomous understanding of compliance and adherence.

I hope I have shown how these interventions in hemophilia care were strongly connected to sociological attachments without developing them into sociological sentimentalities. The interventions in this case were shaped by and produced a figuration of compliance crucially different than those found in the repertoire of distrust or in an autonomy discourse. Such a scholarly approach can thus be productive for overcoming what otherwise tends to become an infertile tension between medical professionals focusing on general compliance enhancement by cognitive training programs and patients having to fit treatment requirements into the complexities of their lives.

In avoiding sociological sentimentality, doctors may turn out to be marginalized by patients, the invisible work of nurses may be suppressed not by clinicians or managers but by their direct colleagues, and patients may be self-reliant to such an extent that it produces unwarranted risks for the safety of other patients: not quite the "usual normative suspects" but a set of empirically unpacked relations that afford crucially different interventions than usually carried out (and critiqued) in compliance-enhancement programs. By probing the practice of hemophilia care and the connections between patients, campsites, doctors, loggers, nurses, and hospital clinics, the practice of hemophilia home treatment turned out to overflow with unexpected normativities to create unforeseen partial connections that helped to produce sociological knowledge about different forms of compliance and different possibilities for its enhancement.

The "tension between the tendency to immerse oneself in the complexities of ethnographic detail" and the "tendency to produce an explicit contribution to a research tradition of theoretical models and empirical findings" (Hess 2001, p. 239) are, therefore, not the main problems in practices of situated intervention. In this approach, the way to *come to* such explicit contributions is *through* immersing oneself in the complexity of practices. Rather than claim that "one can maintain a high standard of descriptive analysis while at the same time providing grounds for making prescriptive recommendations" (ibid., p. 240), I would prefer to say that, in line with the importance of interlocking representing and intervening in the natural sciences, situated intervention in the social sciences implies that *especially through* high standard analysis one can find solid located grounds for experimental interventions, which, in turn, produce sociological knowledge. Having explored the value of situated intervention for both scholarly debates on compliance and for practices of hemophilia home treatment, I now turn to the potential of such research for debates about standardization in health care.

2 Situated Standardization in Hematology and Oncology Care

The Problems of Practice Variation and Evidence-Based Medicine

The idea that lack of standardization is one of the main problems in Western health care systems has, over the past few decades, become commonplace among policy makers and agents of health care improvement. Ever since the publication of John Wennberg and Alan Gittelsohn's (1973) work on local "practice variation" in health care delivery, this has been a major concern for policy makers and professionals alike. Wennberg and Gittelsohn's studies showed that patients with similar diagnoses were treated very differently depending on the hospital they visited or the region they lived in. Regional variation in applying radical mastectomy versus breast-conserving procedures for treating breast cancer ranged from 11 percent to 84 percent among counties and from 6 percent to 84 percent among hospitals (Iscoe et al. 1994). Prostate surgeries varied by factors as high as 8 among geographical locations (Wennberg and Cooper 1999). These were serious causes for concern among quality-of-care researchers, policy makers, and clinicians, especially since the variation could be explained neither by "case-mix" differences (variation in severity of the disease in the population that a hospital or region serves) nor by statistical chance. Once experiments in reducing variation showed a substantial decrease of hospital utilization (Wennberg 1984), policy makers realized that quality-of-care policies and cost-containment policies would both benefit from reducing variations in health care practices. With the cost of health care increasing as a result of the aging of the population, and after repeated efforts to reveal the connection between poor quality and high costs (Committee on Quality of Health Care in America 2001), policy makers and health professionals became convinced that variation is one of the main factors in the quality/cost conundrum.

The advent of evidence-based medicine (EBM) in Western health care systems should be considered in the light of the discovery of this variation problem. Proponents of the self-proclaimed "new paradigm" of medical practice (Evidence-based Medicine Working Group 1992) defined EBM as "the conscientious, explicit, and judicious use of current best evidence in making decisions about the care of individual patients" (Sackett et al. 1996). The paradigm shift they suggested was to move away from the centrality of pathophysiological evidence in the organization and practice of clinical care and toward a privileged epistemological status for epidemiological results (Evidence-based Medicine Working Group 1992; Sackett and Rosenberg 1995). Medical sociologists have argued that one of the flaws in EBM is that it assumes a universal "hierarchy of evidence that consistently places the evidence derived from randomised controlled clinical trials on top" (Goldenberg 2006, p. 2623; cf. Timmermans 2010, p. 309), and ascribe this epistemic hierarchy to the founding fathers of EBM.[1] This hierarchy holds meta-reviews to provide superior credibility over randomized controlled double-blind clinical trials, non-randomized trials, cohort studies, and, at the bottom of the hierarchy, observational studies (Moreira 2007, Timmermans 2010). This epistemological privileging of study outcomes and the absence of clinical experience as an explicit category has led to much criticism of EBM. Much of the criticism has focused on concerns about rationalization of complex care and the potential erasure of individual patients (Mykhalovskiy and Weir 2004). Given the fact that the hierarchy of evidence deals with the *procedural standard* that was followed to produce knowledge (Timmermans and Berg 2003), it says little about the *clinical relevance* of such studies for the care that would best benefit an individual patient. An excessive focus on available evidence rather than on its relevance in the clinical encounter has been polemically defined as "evidence-biased medicine [that uses] evidence in the manner of the fabled drunkard who searched under the streetlamp for his door key because this is where the light was, even though he had dropped the key somewhere else" (Evans 1995, p. 461). In an attempt to remedy the risk of evidence-biased medicine, its founders repeatedly clarified that in EBM clinical experience and scientific evidence were to be treated not as exclusionary but as complementary (Sackett et al. 1996, 2000).

Initially EBM proponents assumed that the proposed paradigm shift would be achieved through changes in medical education. For this reason, the founding publication carried as a subtitle *A New Approach to Teaching the Practice of Medicine* (Evidence-based Medicine Working Group 1992). However, EBM has mostly taken the shape of an *infrastructural* change with the development of clinical practice guidelines (CPGs). According to Stefan Timmermans and Marc Berg (2003, p. 3), the two have become de facto synonyms in medical practice: "In common medical parlance [EBM] mainly denotes the use of *clinical practice guidelines* to disseminate proven diagnostic and therapeutic knowledge." CPGs aim at grounding clinical decision making in the evidence assessed in systematic meta-reviews of randomized clinical trials. The US Institute of Medicine defines CPGs as "systematically developed statements to assist practitioner and patient decisions about appropriate health care for specific clinical circumstances" (Field and Lohr 1990). A plethora of CPGs have been developed and have been made available to large audiences of practitioners by storing them in guideline repositories (Knaapen et al. 2010; Weisz et al. 2007). By 2011, the National Guideline Clearinghouse website of the US Federal Department of Health and Human Services listed more than 7,000 CPGs (Agency for Healthcare Research and Quality 2011). However, the pervasiveness of CPGs seems hardly to have reduced the unwarranted variations in practice that the EBM movement wants to weed out.

EBM, CPGs, ICPs and Minding Their Gaps

In 1981 the American College of Cardiology (ACC) ... began developing clinical practice guidelines to assist in the diagnosis and management of patients with various cardiovascular diseases. ... Although a number of reports have found that implementing practice guidelines leads to improvements in the quality of care delivered, others have found a discouraging lack of guideline implementation and/or impact. Despite the considerable investment in the development and dissemination of guidelines, many studies suggest that a large proportion of eligible patients do not receive the cardiovascular care recommended in guidelines. There continue to be gaps between ideal goals of evidence-based therapy and practice in treatment in several cardiovascular disease states.

The ACC launched the Guidelines Applied in Practice (GAP) Program. ... Key features include building partnerships, flexibility to allow local adaptation, tools derived directly from the guideline, involvement of caregivers across the continuum of care (i.e., not just cardiologists), involvement of patients, use of champions/opinion leaders, and use of data to change behavior and measure effectiveness of the approach.

—http://www.acc.org/qualityandscience/gap/gap_program.htm

Research on standardization of care and clinical guidelines is struggling with ways of bridging what is often referred to as "the gap" between medi-

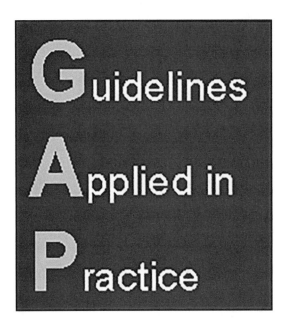

cal quality as defined in clinical guidelines and the practices of care delivery. Treatment methods and procedures that have made it into CPGs are often not encountered when one observes health care work in action. The approximately 50 percent adherence rate of health care professionals to clinical guidelines (Burstin et al. 1999; Grilli and Lomas 1994) is often seen as problematic by health scientists and policy makers alike. Folders of clinical guidelines are often referred to as "paper tigers"; despite their clinical potency, they seldom threaten existing practices in health care work. ICT that draws upon these guidelines is often attributed the power to "address the quality gap in health care by providing automated decision support to clinicians that integrates guideline knowledge with electronic patient data to present real-time, patient-specific recommendations" (Goldstein et al. 2004, p. 368). Yet it is increasingly acknowledged—with a perhaps unintended sense of ironical understatement—that "technical success in implementing decision support systems *may not translate directly* into system use by clinicians" (ibid., emphasis added).

Observations of low adherence rates are often coupled to a sense of bewilderment about variability and to pleas for exploring better strategies for implementing aggregated clinical evidence into the messiness of medical practice (Cabana et al. 1999; Freeman and Sweeney 2001). The discovery of the "implementation problem" of clinical guidelines by the health-care-improvement movement has resulted in a strong interest in studying "factors" that hamper or facilitate their dissemination into medical practice (Grol et al. 1998; Grol 2000; Taylor and Taylor 2004; Grol and Wensing 2004) and in developing rigorously controlled studies to distill these factors—preferably by the methodological gold standard of the randomized controlled trial to ensure evidence-based implementation of EBM.[2] This line of research seems problematic in two ways. First, many years of implementation research show hardly any changes in the way guidelines were integrated with medical practice. Second, the lists of factors for success and failure constructed by such studies are becoming ever longer,[3] thereby providing little guidance to those actively involved in strengthening the relations between medical practices and medical evidence.

This line of reasoning can be characterized as constructing a *moving gap*. Whereas the EBM movement started with the realization that epidemiological evidence was not successful in influencing clinical practice, CPGs were developed to address the knowledge-practice gap. However, practice guidelines seem to face similar gaps in adherence, not to EBM this time, but to the guidelines themselves. They also repeat the same solution of requiring more evidence, but now the evidence that is wanted is about implementation.

One of the problems with research on factors that aid implementation is that it provides "solutions" that leave the privileged epistemological status of aggregated medical knowledge untouched. It merely focuses on *how* practices of health care delivery can be made to "adhere" to the "forefront of medical knowledge" and on how evidence can be "implemented" in patient care (Wensing, Wollersheim, and Grol 2006). Such approaches are at times accompanied by heroic claims that "the best guideline is only a good intention unless it degenerates into clinical care" (Dilts 2005, p. 5881). However, as Sandra Tanenbaum has pointed out (2005, p. 163), succinctly summarizing a series of vigorous controversies around standardization of health care practices, the EBM agenda is a form of epistemological politics, defining which knowledge and which knowers are to be privileged in both policy arenas and consulting rooms. Solutions that fail to deal with these tensions creatively and merely stick to the rhetoric of implementation have therefore proved practically ineffective, politically desensitized, and conceptually problematic. On all these grounds, it therefore seems important to search for practices that help re-conceptualize the problems of standardization and the various modes of knowledge production in health care.

Practitioners of health care improvement are trying to intertwine the practices of care delivery and clinical evidence in the interesting development of integrated care pathways (ICPs).[4] ICPs are defined as "multidisciplinary care management tools which map out chronologically key activities in a healthcare process" (Allen 2009, p. 354). Though pathways were first developed in the 1980s in the American managed care setting, with the main purpose of allowing hospitals to meet the length-of-stay limits imposed by third-party payers (Pinder et al. 2005, p. 761), since the late 1990s they have gained importance not just as ways to implement clinical evidence but also as ways to review it in the light of an equally critical evaluation of the practice of care delivery for which it is to be made relevant. According to Denise Kitchiner (chair of the British National Pathway Association) and her colleague Peter Bundred (1998, p. 147), this critical review of both clinical practice and medical evidence "allows the development of locally agreed guidelines, which are incorporated into the pathway and provide the standard for future routine patient care." "Guidelines," Kitchiner and Bundred continue, "are more likely to succeed if they are developed by those who will be using them. … Analysis of the causes of variation provides valuable information which can be used to improve clinical practice. It also allows clinicians to evaluate the effectiveness of national guidelines at a local level and to collect observational evidence when randomised trials are impractical or unjustified."

The development of pathways can thus be understood as translating practices of health care delivery, as situating clinical evidence in the specificities of care practices, and as articulating other forms of clinically relevant knowledge than the outcomes of randomized controlled trials. This makes their development an interesting site for doing epistemological politics.

Admittedly, such a reading of what Ruth Pinder and colleagues call "the pathway movement" (2005, p. 763) is a generous one. It is equally possible to analyze pathway development as simply aiming at "facilitating the introduction into clinical practice of clinical guidelines and systematic, continuing audit" (Campbell et al. 1998, p. 133). Proponents tend to ascribe almost mythical powers to care pathways. If spread is an indicator of success, then pathways are certainly successful. Kitchiner and Bundred claim that "the rapid increase in the use of pathways supports the recognition that they can provide a powerful tool to facilitate the implementation of locally agreed multidisciplinary guidelines to promote effective clinical care" (1998, p. 147). The strong claims by proponents that such standardization of health care practices can provide impressive increases in efficiency (Evans 1997), effectiveness (Berdick and Humphries 1994), and both patient and professional satisfaction (Ford and Fottler 2000) supports recent policy developments that "include the drive to standardise professional performance in an era troubled by revelations of professional misconduct post-Shipman, and the shift from professional discretion and variability to a more rules-based, audited practice" (Pinder et al. 2005, p. 762). The ICP movement thus increasingly positions pathways as "rationalizing techniques" (Berg 1997, p. 157) for reducing variations in practice.

With its drive to reduce practice variation among health care practitioners, the ICP movement risks becoming just another attempt to "implement" aggregated, pure medical knowledge into the contingent messiness of clinical practice. Pathways have often been "treated uncritically as helpful (and technically neutral) tools rather than embodied practices for routing patients through the system" (Pinder et al. 2005, pp. 762–763), by which members of the ICP movement could exchange an epistemologically political sensitivity for an "over-rationalist and sometimes evangelical" (ibid., p. 763) mode of "modernizing" medical work. This tendency is most obvious in attempts at the beginning of this century to standardize the very practices of developing integrated care pathways. Rather than adopt "a critical and processual understanding of pathways" (ibid.) and their development, the pathway movement has made strong efforts to standardize the development of care paths, which has resulted in highly detailed manuals that lay out a 32-step methodology for designing and implementing a pathway (Vanhaecht and Sermeus 2002).

The ironic consequence is that the success of rigidly developed integrated care pathways has become dependent on their "implementation." The history of epistemological politics that the pathway movement once aimed to reconfigure seems to be repeating itself. Whereas ICPs were developed to address the "implementation problems" produced by an epistemic hierarchy of clinical evidence to which practice has to "adhere," their present conceptualization severely risks reproducing those very problems, thereby moving the knowledge-practice gap further down the implementation line. The discussion of pathways thereby threatens to change from a discussion about the critical analysis of care practice and evidence to one about problems with "implementing" ICPs and assessing their effectiveness (Dy et al. 2003, 2005). Because the preferred method of establishing the results of ICPs is the randomized controlled trial (Marrie et al. 2000), the EBM movement seems to have come full circle. Yet the pathway movement is struck by surprise when it appears that in practice evidence-based implemented pathways are still often used as a "tick box exercise" (Neuberger, Guthrie, and Aaronvitch 2013, p. 3). In view of the recent withdrawal of one of the important care pathways in the United Kingdom after an independent review published under the apt title *More Care, Less Pathway*, and in view of the problematic record of both EBM and CPGs in reducing the dreaded variations in practice, the future of ICPs may not be promising. This future may be all the more troublesome if the assumption that variation is a sign of the lack of accountability of the medical profession remains unchallenged.

ICPs and Standardizing on the Universal/Individual Axis

It would be an overtly pessimistic linear reading of the history of pathway development to claim that the processual understanding of pathwaying has been fully overtaken by the implementation approach. Present initiatives are trying to develop pathways that are to be considered as "complex interventions"[5] whereby pathways should be seen as an *outcome* of a dynamic standardization process, rather than a *starting point* that medical practice has to adhere to. However, such approaches would benefit from a conceptualization of standardization that moves away from the dichotomy of the universal and the particular.

Much of the debate on EBM and the complexities of delivering care centers on this tension that Steve Epstein characterizes as "the abstract debate between universal, standardized approaches to medicine and policy (treating everyone the same as everyone else) and individualized approaches (recognizing the uniqueness of each person)" (2007, p. 14). Epstein suggests that the idea that universal standardization is problematic because of population differences is so widely acknowledged that health care research, health care policy, and health care practice operate in an inclusion-and-difference paradigm. This paradigm aims at "the inclusion of members of various groups generally considered to have been underrepresented previously as subjects in clinical studies" (ibid., p. 6). To produce valid (or monetarily valuable) results, patients with co-morbidity or other complicating factors are generally omitted from randomized controlled trials. For example, some studies on the use of warfarin for atrial fibrillation have gone as far as excluding 97 percent of 18,376 eligible patients (Stroke Prevention in Atrial Fibrillation Investigators 1991), which comes down to "almost all patients in clinical practice" (Gray 2005, p. 66). Furthermore, trial outcomes are subjected to extensive data-cleaning practices to enable the transfer from "dirty data" to reliable evidence (Helgesson 2010). Recognizing that purity of evidence may come at the expense of clinical relevance, the inclusion-and-difference paradigm aims at standardizing not at the level of an abstract universal patient, but at the level of the social group, which is generally operationalized as sex, gender, race, ethnicity, and age. Epstein characterizes this approach as "niche standardization" that proposes "instead of a standard human ... an intersecting set of standard subtypes" (2007, p. 135). Whereas the idea of the standard human is likened to Fordism and its implied universal mass consumer, Epstein compares niche standardization to post-Fordist practices of niche marketing diversified products to well-defined consumer groups. Niche standardization, he proposes, standardizes not at the universal level but at the "'intermediate' level of the categorical group" (ibid., p. 136), and this approach promises a way out of the "polar opposition between leveling and individuation or between universalism and particularism" (ibid.).

The need for niche standardization is challenged by the promise of particularizing standards either through individualized guidelines or personalized medicine. Individualized guidelines avoid the simplistic nature of one-size-fits-all guidelines by using "readily available characteristics from each person to calculate the risk reduction expected from treatment and to identify persons for treatment in ranked order of decreasing expected benefit" (Eddy et al. 2011, p. 637). This combination of assessing risk factors and adjusting recommendations accordingly may help to prevent the dangers of following guideline advice in the cases of multi-morbidity patients, as described in previous studies. Cynthia Boyd and colleagues (2005) have shown that following treatment as prescribed in CPGs could ultimately lead to iatrogenic harm or even mortality. In the treatment of atherosclerosis, recent experimental studies showed, individualized guidelines could prevent 43 percent more myocardial infarctions and strokes for the same cost as treatment according to existing guidelines, while reducing costs by 67 percent for the same benefit obtained by adhering to the same guidelines as published by the Joint National Committee on Prevention, Detection, Evaluation, and Treatment of High Blood Pressure (Eddy et al. 2011; Owens 2011). This does not merely point to the promise of individualized guidelines; it also challenges the idea that professionals' present low rates of adherence to guidelines are problematic per se. As a clinician commenting on a *New York Times* editorial said of publications on these initiatives, "You know what 'individualized guideline' is—the art of practicing medicine." This statement seems to be confirmed by Marc Oertle and Roland Bal's 2010 study of the *reasons* professionals have for deviating from recommendations on drug prescription in a guideline for chronic heart failure. In a quantitative part of their study, Oertle and Bal corrected non-adherence for factors such as the most important clinical contraindication (renal insufficiency) and influencing co-morbidity such as chronic obstructive pulmonary disease and hypotension, and found that this correction raised the commonly used guideline adherence index (GAI) to 60 percent. Further qualitative study through repeated interviews with physicians on their clinical judgment in particular cases showed that additional correction was needed for factors such as rapidly changing symptoms, errors in diagnostic data, or uncertainty due to recent diagnoses. Such correction led to a GAI score of 90 percent, with clinicians explaining their actions for example as follows:

This patient was just confronted with the diagnosis of [chronic heart failure]. We do not know for how long his heart did not work well and I don't know how he will react on our drugs. What should I do now? Should I give him every recommended drug in the guideline or should I step up with the most important ones and look how he reacts? The guideline does not tell you that (ibid., p. 4).

Thus, although niche standardization is under pressure from the promise of individualized guidelines, the experiments aimed at redeeming this promise are creating unwieldy computational risk-adjustment models that at best may come close to prevailing clinical practice, rather than providing solutions for *problematic* forms of non-adherence to guidelines.

The need for niche standardization is similarly challenged by the new science of pharmacogenomics, which, according to its proponents, "will permit truly individualized drug therapy according to each person's specific genetic polymorphisms" (Epstein 2007, p. 225). In personalized medicine, dosage and drug specificity are tailored to the specific genetic characteristics of individual patients. However, such individualization of drugs may not be interesting to pharmaceutical companies, since (to quote Troy Duster) "Individuals are not a market. Groups are a market."[6] Consequently, pharmacogenomics and individualized guidelines are questionable long-term solutions.

Pharmacogenomics has been called a "promissory science" (Hedgecoe 2004) rather than a nearby reality. Much the same applies to individualized guidelines, which are presented as "the way of medicine in the future" (David M. Eddy, cited in Chen 2011) but which may fall short of that prediction because of problematic assumptions. Epstein (2007, p. 227) therefore proposes that the hype and hope of individualization should not get in the way of crucial questions about "what happens at the interim" of the standardization debate. And this is where he positions niche standardization.

In some ways, CPGs and ICPs are already forms of niche standardization. They are geared toward the treatment of specific groups defined by a common diagnosis. The way forward that seems the preferred option for proponents of the inclusion-and-difference paradigm is to further specify the niches by subdividing diagnostic groups in social groups. A given range of factors that could be clinically relevant is, however, much wider than the categories of sex, gender, race, ethnicity, and age that niche standardization in the inclusion-and-difference-paradigm seems to address. The warfarin study mentioned above contained no fewer than 24 exclusion criteria, ranging from dementia to a short life expectancy due to metastatic cancer (Stroke Prevention in Atrial Fibrillation Investigators 1991, p. 528). Thus, clinically relevant niche standardization would soon end up relatively close to the promissory practice of individualized medicine. This problem may come from the fact that niche standardization by group profiling still operates on the universal/individual axis, while it mainly focuses on the level of granularity of the standard. Since niche standardization is "located in some sense between individuality and universality" (Epstein 2007, p. 279), it may be unable to overcome the tensions this dichotomy produces and thereby fail to be of real use in helping to prevent the pathway movement from reproducing the very knowledge-practice gap it set out to bridge. To explore an alternative type of standardization that bypasses the universal-individual dichotomy, I propose to take inspiration from the study of street patterns.

Situated Standardization as Bypassing the Universal/Individual Axis

In an attempt to analyze the relative efficiency of various types of cities, Italian physicists have shown that the additional distance one has to cover to get from any particular point in a city to any other point in that city is strikingly similar for cities with very different characteristics (Cardillo et al. 2006). Because one cannot travel in a straight line, but has to move along roads and streets and avoid buildings, the extra distance needed to get from A to B can be captured in the "minimum spanning tree." Through their analysis of the street patterns in 20 cities around the world, Cardillo and colleagues have shown that the minimum spanning tree in a relatively unstructured medieval city such as Ahmedabad (figure 2.1) is strikingly similar to that of a grid-style city such as New York (figure 2.2). This means that when getting around in New York one has to span, on average, the same distance as when getting around in the incrementally developed streets of Ahmedabad. I suggest that this counter-intuitive finding is illustrative of the polar oppositions of universal standardization and individualized medicine. The striking similarities between Ahmedabad and New York may be illuminating both for the potential limitations of celebrating complexity and for those of rationalizing medical work.

Similar results for the spatial arrangements of other cities, particularly Paris (figure 2.3), are worth exploring. Paris is especially interesting because Cardillo and colleagues qualify it as "hybrid," meaning that it has some of the qualities of New York and some of those of Ahmedabad. Paris can

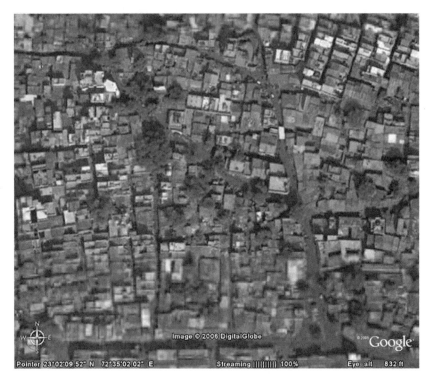

Figure 2.1
Ahmedabad.

be seen as an ancient city with a substantial "organic" development, but some parts of it were thoroughly structured in the nineteenth century by Hausmannization, which involved the development of *grande* connections through *allées* and *boulevards*. And, as the physicists have calculated, such a city has *a far lower minimum spanning tree* than any of its more homogeneous counterparts. Getting from A to B in a hybrid city requires a shorter journey than in either a medieval or a grid-style city. The hybrid qualities of Paris thereby provide an interesting metaphor for what I call *situated standardization* of medical practice.

Situated standardization privileges neither complexity nor standardization as a harbinger of good medical practice. It tries to empirically elucidate specific issues in care delivery so that an assessment can be made of which aspects of the organization of care should be given space and which aspects should be standardized. This situates the "solution" of particular standardization attempts in specifically articulated issues. It makes standardization neither an *a priori* solution (which would lead to grid-style medical work)

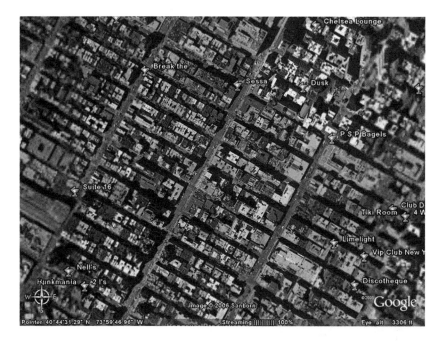

Figure 2.2
New York.

nor a solution merely open to the criticism that it isn't sufficiently sensitive to the complexities of prevailing work practices (which would lead to celebrating complexity while ignoring the issues at stake). Situated standardization is a located and therefore accountable attempt to address specific issues in the delivery of health care (cf. Suchman 2002). In the remainder of this chapter, I explore the role of situated intervention in the social sciences for strengthening the processual approach to standardization.

Situated Standardization for Hematology and Oncology Care

The hemophilia care center on which I focused in chapter 1 was part of a large hematology/oncology outpatient clinic and day care treatment center in which chemotherapy and blood transfusions were administered. Because of the situated-intervention project on hemophilia care that was underway there, the management of this outpatient clinic, consisting of medical professionals and health care managers, invited our institute to analyze the problems they faced in the organization of care. Because of such problems as long waiting times for diagnostic procedures (particularly CT and MRI

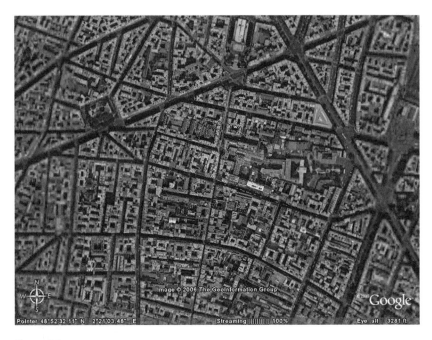

Figure 2.3
Paris.

scans) and periodic overcrowding in the day care treatment center, they faced great difficulties in delivering the care they wanted to deliver to their patients, and they were struggling to guarantee that all trials could be carried out precisely as prescribed in trial protocols. In emergency situations, patients were receiving chemotherapy while sitting up on stools rather than while reclining in an adjustable chair, something that was seen as an unacceptable safety risk. During my initial three-month study, I used a combination of ethnographic and quantitative approaches to analyze the problems patients and care workers faced on the ward.

It turned out that the outpatient clinic and treatment center had doubled its number of patients in just three years. Staff members were making a huge effort to meet pressing needs but increasingly faced difficulties they could not overcome. As a consequence, the curative aspect of care prevailed over other aspects that were not directly relevant to the continuation of treatment.

Mrs. Durga, a lady in her late fifties, enters the treatment center nervously. She looks around uncertainly. Clearly she is coming here for the first time and does not know the way yet.

Gina, one of the nurses in the day care treatment center, invites Mrs. Durga to sit in one of the available chairs and explains how to adjust it to suit herself: "It's handy to first lift the armrest and then get in. That way the chair won't be too high. And you can get out that way as well. Soon you will have to stay still for your course for four hours. At the end of this room, around the corner, there is a restroom. It would be good if you used it now, then you won't have to walk with the drip afterwards. You'll be getting Taxol in a bit. Have you had a chemotherapy course here before?"

"No, not here ... yet," says Mrs. Durga.

"I thought you'd never had a course before," Gina continues.

"Well, I did ... When was it?... I think I already had ... one, perhaps two years ago." Mrs. Durga seems somewhat confused.

Gina quickly explains the steps of the treatment. The first bag, then the next, something against nausea, something against reactions to the treatment.

It appears that Mrs. Durga can't follow all the steps. "Well, fine," she jokes. "If I start convulsing, I'll let you know."

"You may laugh now, but it really can happen," says Gina. "You could have a reaction, a convulsion in fact. But it's not likely."

Mrs. Durga is visibly shocked. Gina emphasizes once more that there is only a minor chance of such a bad reaction. After this, Mrs. Durga meekly goes to the restroom, and on her return Gina inserts the chemotherapy drip in her arm.

Afterwards Gina sighs to me. "Dear o dear. ... Before, we always had an orientation chat with new patients coming for the first time. We had a small, separate room in the back for that. But we had to install a bed for treatment in there. [The center has] grown so much that we can't deliver some very basic forms of care. On top of that, when you realize that the surgery hours are completely overbooked, you know there is no time for their questions either, I sometimes wonder what kind of care we are actually delivering here."

Since the introduction to the center now took place at the start of the treatment session, and since a public setting is not the most suitable place to discuss private matters of concern, the introduction focused strongly on practical issues, and even those were barely explained to patients.

Because of the overcrowded surgery hours with many more patient visits than available appointment slots, and the resulting workload at the appointments desk in the treatment center, the definition of good work seemed to have shifted from caring for individual needs to keeping up the high pace. "Good staff members" meant efficient staff members, but even among these hard-working professionals, and despite good intentions, tensions were running high, and at times they led to direct confrontations between the physicians and the assistants who managed their appointments. In one case an upset hematologist refused to see a patient added as the seventeenth appointment in a surgery hour with twelve slots. The assistant had not checked with him whether the patient's case was really that urgent, and this crossed a line for this overburdened doctor.

As a center for tertiary care, the outpatient clinic dealt with a substantial number of patients visiting for a second opinion. The diagnostics conducted in the hospital that was treating them were often not available. Max Kampman, an oncologist, sighed when he said "Sometimes you can only hope that patients come in with their own scans." New patients referred for thrombosis and hemostasis needed to have diagnostic tests to establish hereditary predisposition, but these tests were ordered during, rather than before, the intake consultation. Since this group of patients made up about 42 percent of all new diagnoses on this ward, this led to hundreds of unnecessary follow-up visits, which increased the pressure on the surgery hours. The time needed to see patients differed markedly. Discussions about whether or not to start a new series of chemotherapy treatments took far longer than visits by lymphoma patients who needed only to have their blood values checked to see if their regular dose of chemotherapy could be administered. Because of delays in the room where patients gave blood samples, such blood values were not always readily available. Blood samples were taken in the order of patients' arrival rather than in the order in which they would see the clinician, and since many patients calculated buffer time to avoid traffic and arrived at the hospital at the same time, early mornings were busy and lab results for early scheduled patients often not available. Waiting for a patient's lab results was one of the most annoying experiences for physicians. Peter Linden, whom we also met in chapter 1, remarked "It's so frustrating, because this way you can only run *late*; you can't ever run *early.*" Yvo Jacobs, another doctor avoided frustration by making best use of the waiting time, and remarked "I always bring in work when I have surgery."

In a period of five months, hematologists had worked 680 hours of surgery, 170 more than the 510 planned hours. They had 34 additional surgery hours each month, an additional 33 percent, and on average clinics ran 51 minutes late. On top of the regular clinics conducted by staff members, doctors in training ran an emergency surgery in case patients showed up with urgent problems, such as high fever and other reactions to treatment, or a rapid decline in their health. My analysis of these clinics, however, showed that not all the time was spent on urgent cases. This emergency clinic had turned into three to four hours extra hours of surgery on most days, adding up to about 53 hours a month. One of the most striking findings was that new patients were also given appointments in the emergency hours of doctors in training. These patients were generally referred to a tertiary cancer hospital, since they could no longer be treated properly in the general hospital, but now they ended up being seen by a doctor who was *in training* to work in a general hospital. Staff members were well aware of the undesirability of this situation, but were also firm about not increasing the access time to their ward, as having to wait for access to tertiary cancer care was seen as unacceptable.

Among oncologists there was no such mismatch between the amount of surgery scheduled and the amount delivered. Here, however, there was a substantial difference between individual oncologists and the way they conducted their surgery. Table 2.1, which summarizes a few outliers, is based on the standard time slots of 20 minutes for a return visit, 45 minutes for a new patient, and 5 minutes for a telephone consult.

One of the most noteworthy consequences of generating these overviews was that they seemed indispensable to creating credibility in a medical setting where blood values, tumor markers and trial outcomes defined much of what counted and mattered. Physicians eagerly wrote down the figures I presented, and this created legitimacy for some of the changes I proposed for the ward. The importance of metrication was due in part to the legitimacy it created and in part to medical professionals' trust in numbers (Porter 1995), which made such overviews part of the "ingenious solutions" the social sciences have to come up with to face "the problem of how to become interesting enough for practices to care about" (Jensen and Lauritsen 2005, p. 72). According to Jensen and Lauritsen (ibid., p. 73), "it is doubtful if either dry sociological monographs or elliptical reflexive writing are up to this task." But metrication was also crucial to creating

Table 2.1
Large variation in oncology surgery hours.

Scheduled duration	Number of patients	Type of visits	Running early or late	Deviation from norm
4:00 h	17	17 return	0:00 h	−1:40 h
4:00 h	15	14 return, 1 phone	−0:50 h	−1:35 h
3:45 h	12	7 return, 5 phone	3:00 h	3:55 h
2:20 h	12	10 return, 2 phone	4:50 h	3:40 h

various partial connections needed to change the practice once this interest was gained.

The overviews of hours spent on surgery and types of patients seen were not difficult to produce. It turned out that a previous ward manager had instituted the practice of "closing" surgery hours, which meant that doctors' assistants registered the actual start and end times at the end of the morning clinic and at the end of the afternoon clinic. However, new management had never showed much interest in the overviews this practice could produce. That caused dismay among members of the support staff in the IT department. They had developed management reporting schemes to show the delays of clinics, but were frustrated that management was not using such useful features but did voice many complaints about the somewhat dated IT systems the hospital used. They were therefore eager to help again when I showed interest in the possibilities the IT system *did* offer. With some tinkering with the reporting possibilities, IT support staff produced useful overviews, meanwhile preparing the grounds for more regular reporting schemes.

What I wish to indicate with this mundane example of gathering data on surgery hours is that the analysis of issues on the ward was not merely a "design phase" of thinking up solutions. It was a way to get involved in the issues at the hematology/oncology outpatient clinic. This investigation proved crucial to creating partial connections to various elements of the ward, such as doctors, the planning module of the hospital information system, nurses, the hospital's IT department, doctors' assistants, strategies for working together with hospitals in the region, secretaries, plans for renovating the ward, hospital management, and the finance and control department. It was also an opportunity to link the ward to various practices to which it was not yet allied, including the children's hospital that was doing triage in a new consultancy-developed way that the management there was about to dismantle, an oncology ward in another university hospital that had developed a planning system for its treatment center that was yielding good results, and sociological literature and conference talks on standardization.

Still, after this first phase, I wrote a formal proposal for changes that could be experimented with on the ward. I concluded that the problems I encountered included three important issues: the strong variability of the weekly workload, the absence of a planning system for the treatment center of the ward, and the clearly overcrowded surgery hours of both hematologists and oncologists. The implied solutions were, thus, reducing variability by shifting surgery hours around to find a better distribution over the week, developing a planning system for the treatment center to ensure that a critical resource would be put at center stage in the planning of activities, and opening up space in the surgery hours of the doctors.

The aim of this chapter is not to give a complete account of the project and the interventions that we experimented with. However, it is worth noting that some definitions of the issues of this ward were explicitly not taken into account in the conclusions of the analysis. One such definition was that, in order to prevent chaos at the appointments counter, the tasks should be divided into front-office and back-office activities. Doctors' assistants should either carry out front-office activities, and be available for patients, or else do back-office activities in a separate room. Henk Hulst, the unit manager, proposed this approach, inspired by the customer relationship management (CRM) promoted in articles in management journals (e.g., Chase and Tansik 1983). However, my ethnographic observations showed that the only way doctors' assistants could manage the peak loads on the ward was by noticing when a colleague was about to fall behind in serving patients and then helping him or her. I claimed that separating the activities of doctors' assistants without first addressing the causes of peaks in the working load would have a detrimental effect on the work flow. Generally, STS researchers are not best known as authorities on organizational issues,[7] but this statement seemed to be legitimized by the ethnographic research and by my position at a management institute.

The problems and the solutions we agreed upon were the outcome of all the interactions that had taken place in the preceding phase. When my analysis was accepted, medical coordinators were positioned "in the lead" of the project by their appointment as chairs of the working groups for hematology and oncology. These multi-professional groups included staff members, nurses, doctors' assistants, research nurses, the management of the secretaries, the operational manager of the ward, and me. We met once a week to discuss the progress of the project and to work out pathwaying options for the large majority of patients. The set-up with multi-professional working groups with the medical coordinators as chairs made my role one of "acting with," which meant that I had to give up some of my freedom to propose interventions and get them accepted. It also involved a different distribution of the project's ownership and its interventions, which proved crucial both during the project and after its completion.

The experiments in this project contributed to the development of a conceptual approach to standardization of care that aimed at overcoming the universal/individual dichotomy. I worked on the experiments together with Marc Berg and Roland Bal, my colleagues at the Department of Health

Policy and Management. The aim of this approach was to change health care organizations from their unit-based organizational structure (outpatient clinic, laboratories, radiology department, clinical departments) to a process-based organization focused on the flow of patients through health care organizations.[8] Conceptually, this approach to standardizing health care practice draws on the process-based focus of care pathways, and moves away from the standardization of trajectories of individual patients and the process of decision making by individual specialists. Rather than trying to standardize individual patient trajectories, which are bound to have highly specific demands and which may vary as a result of delays in chemotherapy courses, standardization is situated on an *aggregated level*—that is, in *specific issues patient groups face* because they have to make use of the same resource. Regarding such issues, it turns out, trajectories display substantial similarities. Whereas individual patient trajectories are inherently unpredictable, analyzing the trajectory for groups of patients makes certain elements of them more predictable and allows for care to be organized accordingly. Even if the variability of singular care trajectories precludes the planning of specific steps for individual patients, it is possible to assess how often a particular problematic event is likely to occur for a group of patients and to make sure the organization is ready to meet this demand.

A good example of such an event is the emergency CT scan. If an oncology patient has a relapse, such scans are needed to assess whether continuing the present treatment is a sensible step or whether the treatment should be adjusted or even abandoned. Though it is impossible to assess for individual patients whether or when they will have a relapse, every week some patients are bound to face such difficulties. So, rather than booking every slot in the CT schedule because one cannot plan for the unexpected for individual patients, it is possible to have CT time available for emergencies by either working with dedicated emergency slots or by creating direct access to the radiology department. This capacity can then be assigned on a last-minute basis to individual patients. Another example is how patients make collective use of the surgery hours of hematologists and oncologists. The intensity of treatment in tertiary oncology is bound to result in delays in treatment, because of blood values that do not permit a course of chemotherapy to be administered. In that case, patients must return after a week to see if they have recovered sufficiently to get the course at that time. Such dynamics cannot be organized on an individual level, but it is certainly possible to standardize buffer slots in surgery hours to prevent instances in which a next-week return leads to an almost impossible quest for a new appointment. This also requires space to be created in surgery hours, for example by eliminating unnecessary follow-up visits for hemostasis patients by ordering their genetic diagnostics in advance—obviously to the advantage of those patients as well as to the advantage of patients who could have used their appointment slot for a rescheduled visit. This principle of reducing follow-up through better preparation of surgery also applies to other diagnostic trajectories.

Traditionally, and for good reasons, STS researchers would be skeptical of a standardization initiative that claims to sweep aside the problems of the complexity of patient trajectories by claiming to address the issue at an aggregate level. Often the politics of aggregation is bound to a claim to serve everyone better, whereas in fact it accomplishes this ambition at a high expense for those marginalized or excluded (Star 1991b). Such criticism, however, has mainly been directed to the type of standardization that health-care-improvement researchers working on reducing ward-access times of patients have called "carve out" (Silvester et al. 2004), which is the practice of reserving capacity for specific categories of patients—typically financially interesting patients, such as those undergoing cataract surgery or hip replacement. The problem with reserving capacity for such specific patient groups is that the patients who do not fit in the category or do not fit the assumed standard are, de facto, excluded from the arrangement. Such privileging certain patients at the expense of others makes it highly questionable whether the overall situation improves. Yet this is what much of pathway development is about: the development of pathways for specific patient groups, rather than for capacity units that a number of groups need to use. The difference between standards that affect smaller groups and standards that effect the entire population points to the important difference between niche and situated standardization. While standardization at the niche level of patient groups risks marginalizing other niches and thereby producing a problem of the representativeness and legitimacy of the privileged niche, standardization situated in specific issues in the organization of care for all patients using a certain facility does not have to face the problem of marginalizing other niches. Fortunately for patients that do not fit the proposed niches, many medical-improvement researchers working on the logistics of health care and reducing access times share the STS hesitation to niche standardization. They propose a logistic alternative to the problematic idea of ever increasing the number of categories simply by developing more pathways. In contrast, they propose working with "advanced" or "direct access" (Murray and Berwick 2003). This approach does not separate urgent from non-urgent patients to treat the latter sooner at the expense of the former. It tries to undo the extra work the management of such categories involves by treating patients as quickly as possible and desirable.

An important principle of this approach to developing standardized care trajectories is that they are no longer the *point of departure* for the organizational change and implementation that follow the design phase. They are the *outcome* of the project as a whole. How care trajectories would look did not become apparent until we were experimentally exploring which organizational interventions were feasible. The ongoing aim was to avoid designing pathways that would then need implementation, which meant we would have re-created "implementation problems." By conceptualizing care trajectories as an outcome of an experimental standardization process, it proved possible to "prevent" implementation and its problems.

Since this approach was the conceptual starting point of the research, the working groups pursued situating solutions by sketching flow charts for all relevant patient groups to see how they related to the issues met at the outpatient clinic and treatment center. Figures 2.4 and 2.5 are examples of such charts. Because I wanted to avoid the "carve out" issue mentioned above, and because I wanted standardization to have consequences for all patients of the ward rather than for a select group, we sketched charts for a large majority of patients.

Because the hematologists registered all initial diagnoses, we could easily estimate that we would need twelve standardized care pathways to cover 69 percent of the patients, which we decided would be a large enough group to seriously affect the work of the ward. Therefore, we sketched pathways for patients with Hodgkin's lymphoma, patients under the age of 65 with non-Hodgkin's lymphoma, patients over 65 with non-Hodgkin's lymphoma, patients with recurring follicular non-Hodgkin's lymphoma, patients with general chronic lymphatic leukemia, patients with chronic lymphatic leukemia (as part of a trial for new monoclonal antibody medication), patients under 65 with multiple myeloma, patients over 65 with multiple myeloma, and patients undergoing hemostasis, thrombosis, and hemophilia treatment, and patients undergoing Phase I/II trials. Only the hemophilia pathway was a somewhat inconsequential description of an existing practice, since it reflected the improvement project that was the focus of chapter 1 above. Since oncologists did not maintain a register, we had to estimate the number of care pathways needed to cover the large majority of their patients. This seemed possible through six additional trajectories: those for

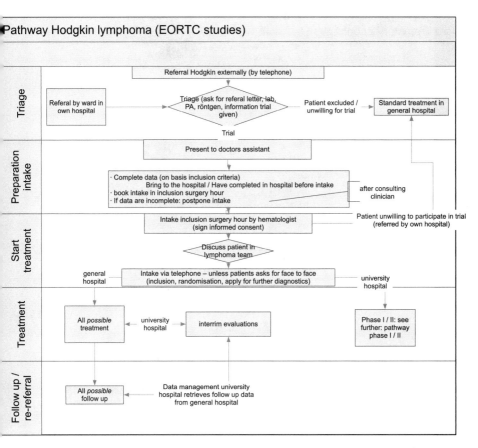

Figure 2.4
Care trajectory for Hodgkin's lymphoma.

bladder carcinoma, colon carcinoma, esophagus carcinoma, ovary carcinoma, testis carcinoma, and Phase I trials.

Most striking in comparison with other forms of integrated care pathways is the relative simplicity of figure 2.4. Whereas ICPs tend to be highly detailed documents and charts that can easily be up to 20 pages in length, including time-task matrices that indicate precisely what action each professional is to undertake at each and every moment of treatment, none of the pathway flow charts we made in this project were more than one page long. Rather than standardize all aspects of (for example) the niche of patients with Hodgkin's lymphoma, we focused the standardized pathways on particular issues that were problematic for patients and professionals on the ward.

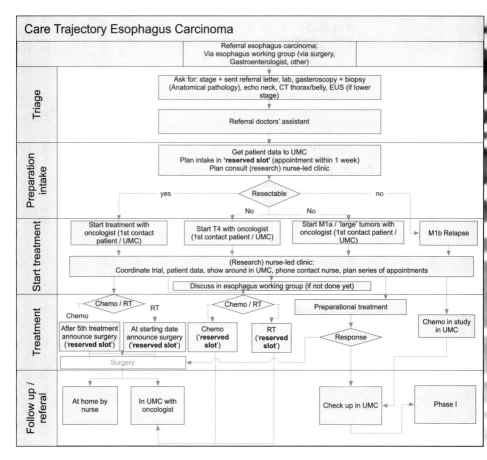

Figure 2.5
Care trajectory for esophagus carcinoma.

Situating Standardization and Flexibility

One problem was the preparation of patient intake. During the initial phase of this project, return visits occurred often because the diagnostics needed to make the first visit useful were not available, either because the material had not yet arrived at the university hospital or because the tests had not been ordered before the visit. Well-prepared intakes could remove substantial pressure on the overburdened surgery hours and release the workload at the appointments counter, as it would be easier to find a slot for patients who really did need follow-up visits. We therefore focused on preparing the intake so that doctors' assistants would be equipped to complete all required diagnostics and background data that would ensure a meaningful intake consult with the hematologist. Time for this was found by stopping the practice of binding printed results into paper records (still kept alongside electronic medical records), since these results were already available in digital form and using paper was merely force of habit.[9]

Not only were doctors' assistants preparing the visits more thoroughly; they were also entitled to postpone an intake visit if data were incomplete. This was done to avoid inefficient visits that put a strain on both patients and the ward. To stop this from leading to unacceptable delays for urgent visits, the assistants always had to ask the consulting physician whether a postponement would be permitted. This generally led to a final check as to whether the data really could not be obtained—for example, by sending an urgent reminder email to the referring specialist in the general hospital.

Another important aspect of the hematological pathways was that they formalized a developing collaboration with general hospitals during the treatment phase. Specialized nurses functioned as data managers for trials. This made it practicable for much of the treatment to be delivered in the general hospital, closer to the patient's home, without jeopardizing the reliability of trial data. It also reduced the number of follow-up visits in the university hospital, an aspect of standardizing care paths that I will return to shortly.

For the oncological pathways there was an equal focus on intake preparation; however, because fewer diagnoses were treated, general hospitals were already well instructed on what the university hospital needed to start treatment. Still, staff members found poorly prepared intakes frustrating, even when patients were not aware of the uncoordinated process. "I usually find a way out if I don't have the right data," Hayo van Doorn, a junior oncologist explained. "I tell patients that we always discuss each and every one of them in our tumor working group. People like to hear this, though it is utter nonsense of course. If I had all the data I needed, I would discuss it on the spot with my supervisor and could decide on a course of action."

Other doctors said that they felt stressed by the idea that patients often were sufficiently well informed that they could ask questions to find out whether data were missing.

Besides improving the preparation of intake visits, we focused on long delays for CT scans and radiotherapy, for access to the surgery department, and for access to the operating theater. Because these problems exceeded the limits of the project at the hematology/oncology outpatient clinic, the solutions we chose (for example, arranging dedicated slots for all the patients from the oncology clinic at the radiology department) were closer to niche standardization. This way the niche was defined at the highest level of aggregation feasible in the project, though undoubtedly there was a risk that it would lead to problems for other patient groups of the university hospital. Still, an important difference was that the assistants on duty at the appointments counter could book appointments for CT scans that they would have done anyway, but without the delays they now experienced.

Many discussions about the way care trajectories were developed centered on various versions of the flow charts. They proved to be interesting experimental devices in the delicate process of articulating specific issues. At a certain time, different versions of flow charts were used to explicate a difference in practice among medical professionals. The hematologists had a lively discussion about what to do with the late follow-up of some forms of treatment. Follow-up of lymphoma treatment is life-long, because patients always risk facing a relapse or a new episode. For that reason, many slots in the hematologists' surgery hours were filled with late follow-ups, which of course caused friction in a setting characterized by a scarcity of slots. "It's because of *this 20 percent* of my surgery hours," Lonneke Blank, a senior hematologist said, holding her hands about 10 centimeters out from her own neck, "that I cannot see a patient referred with a neck *this* thick." She questioned whether the follow-up of these patients was really part of her job, since it stopped her from seeing patients in acute need. A swollen neck indicates swollen glands, which are typically seen in severe cases of lymphatic cancer. Since nearly all patients with severe lymphatic cancer are tertiary referrals, they had nowhere else to go, in contrast with patients just coming in for late follow-up. She agreed with my suggested solution: to send the follow-up patients back to the hospital that had initially referred them and said this was possible, since data managers of the university hospital were visiting regional hospitals regularly to check completion of research data in the medical records kept there. This practice of gathering follow-up data from the records of referring hospitals was already in place for some trials and could be extended to all late follow-ups. This way, she claimed, she could see more patients needing highly specialized care and patients could receive their follow-up in a hospital much closer to where they lived.

However strong the arguments in favor of this change may seem, Hans van Barneveld, the head of the department—the person commissioning the project—held a very different view. He stated that handing over late follow-up to referring hospitals would jeopardize the success of the university hospital in studying late complications such patients face. He saw this as a serious risk to the academic duty of the organization, which he saw as undesirable from the point of view of both care delivery and scientific research. In response, and to facilitate this discussion, I made two competing flow charts of care trajectories. One was similar to figure 2.4 above; the other, shown here as figure 2.6, showed the option of re-referral of patients for late follow-up to general hospitals. Also, further metrication was needed. With Lonneke Blank, the hematologist who favored handing

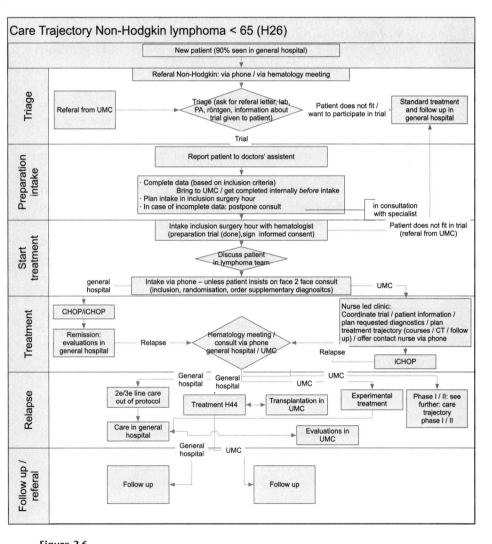

Figure 2.6
Care trajectory for non-Hodgkin's lymphoma, with follow-up in both the general hospital and the university hospital.

over late follow-up to general hospitals, I calculated how big a percentage of the surgery hours was spent on late follow-up of large trials that could be handed over to the referring hospitals with minimal risk of missing late complications. The result we arrived at was approximately 11 percent of all consultations. She had first estimated 20 percent, but to avoid a heated debate we differentiated between patients for whom she was certain that no late complications would be missed and those for whom there were still minor risks, and that lowered the percentage. Finally, I calculated how many extra surgery hours would have to be staffed in case the hematologists decided to consider all late follow-up an integral part of their treatment work.

Before these calculations, the discussion around this topic was taking place at a relative distance from the practice of delivering care. The medical staff held meetings to decide on their strategy in the absence of nurses and operational management. This seemed to result in a somewhat content-biased decision that management merely had to "carry out" rather than be involved in. Organizational consequences of clinical strategy decisions were generally not translated into consequences for the supporting staff and organization—leading to many "implementation problems." It was not easy to overcome this practice of decision making and in stead relate content of care decisions to their organizational consequences of overcrowded surgery hours and stressed personnel; neither I nor the management of the outpatient clinic was welcome at the staff meeting that discussed these issues. Through the experimental introduction of contradicting flow charts and calculations of the number of patients and the time needed for late follow-up in this session, I tried to ally organizational knowledge with the decision making of medical professionals. However, this did not lead to anything resembling more "rationalized" decision making in regard to late follow-up.

After the charts and calculations had been discussed at the hematology staff meeting, when I checked with Lonneke Blank what the outcome of the meeting was, she said that it had led to a brief discussion but that the real (and heated) topic of the meeting had been the staff's boycott of a newly introduced administrative system for registering diagnosis-related groups (DRGs)—a kind of product code—for each patient. This boycott was not targeted at the system itself, but was used as leverage to try to increase the salaries of academic junior doctors, since the hematologists saw all their good young colleagues move on to general and teaching hospitals where salaries were substantially higher. The boycott by university hospitals caused much anxiety for Hans van Barneveld, the departmental head, who wanted the registration to be complete for budgetary and academic reasons. Registration was both connected to billing insurance companies and needed for managing clinical trials. The rising tension dominated the meeting. Why the hematologists did not want anyone looking over their shoulders during the staff meeting was understandable.

General staff meetings on strategic issues were rare. Perhaps because of the tension that was in the air about the boycott of the registration system, the sensitive issue of the late follow-up did not reappear on the agenda. However, when I interviewed the hematologists at the end of the project, Fieny Huijer, one of the senior hematologists, said:

The discussion as to whether late follow-up should be carried out here or in the periphery may not be properly closed, in fact it may never have been brought up for open discussion. But as a matter of fact, most of us now refer those patients back [to the general hospital]. Lonneke, Hayo, and I certainly don't keep those patients for follow-up. After a few years we simply send them back. But you can't do this all at once. You have to announce it two or three times. If you were to suddenly send them away, they'd be standing on your doorstep after three months with all kinds of complaints. They become far too insecure then.

And Lonneke Blank said: "I simply send them back, even though the discussion is not closed. I just want space in my surgery hours."

It is hard to imagine how it could have been beneficial to formalize this practice in a decision about the design of a standardized care trajectory that would have to be implemented. It would merely have polarized the discussion of a sensitive matter of medical content, whereas more implicit standards, with a settlement for what seemed practically feasible at minimal risk, proved more fruitful for addressing the organizational issues of the ward. Without further exploring the differences in late follow-up as a separate category for patients who could be seen in a general hospital, we developed an indicator for the return rate per doctor, measuring the ratio of patients coming for the first time relative to patients coming for other visits. Because there was a separate code for follow-up visits in the surgery agendas, the IT department could easily help generate this indicator, whereas a more detailed indicator about referring back low-risk patients for follow-up to general hospitals would have been nearly impossible to generate. Though this resulted in a standard that left space for not referring late-follow-up patients back to the hospitals that initially referred them for tertiary care, it helped some hematologists who were responsible for a substantial number of surgery hours. It showed that the level at which return rates were assessed was part of the politics of standardization. A *less specific* standard was *more productive* in addressing the problems at hand.

Situated Standardization and Its Consequences

After about a year of pathwaying around specific issues, the situation was quite different. Intake preparation was carefully done by doctors' assistants, who were supported by referral messages they would send to referring hospitals, checklists for the required data per diagnosis, and contact data for most referring specialists in the region that enabled the assistants to follow up on referral messages. In collaboration with the IT staff, we developed a "demo" of a module in the hospitals' electronic patient record that was intended to facilitate preparation work and to ensure the availability of test results and CT scans during the intake visits. (See figure 2.7.)

Referring specialists from general hospitals began getting used to the new practice on the hematology/oncology ward, and to being contacted by the doctors' assistants with requests for additional information on the

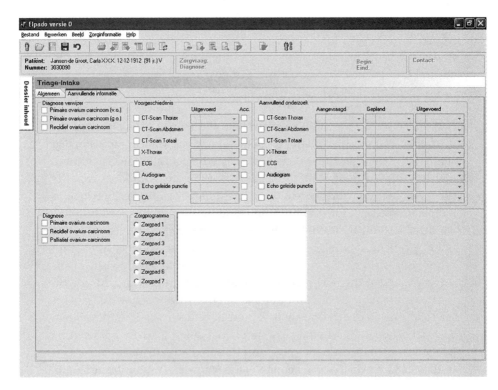

Figure 2.7
Module for preparing intake visits.

patients they referred. "Even today," said Ton Heger, a physician's assistant, "I was called back by a specialist in training [from a referring teaching hospital] about the message. He was wondering what on earth it was all about. The moment I explained it, he immediately sent me this whole stack of files."

Clinics were still running late, but limiting the number of follow-up visits and the number of unnecessary extra visits due to poorly prepared intake reduced the time surgery hours ran late by 53 percent, from an initial average of 51 minutes to 24 minutes by the end of the project. The surgery hours for emergency visits that were run by junior doctors and that had turned into regular surgery hours of almost four hours on most days was reduced to 2.43 hours. Though the aim was never to reduce these surgery hours to zero, as there would always be emergency visits that tend to take longer than regular visits, this reduction benefited the junior doctors, who now had more time to prepare their regular surgery. New patients were no longer booked in the extra surgery hours; now there was time for them in their own newly installed surgery. That was made possible by the time freed up by reducing return visits.

Although the improvements were substantial, and although both professionals and patients noticed the difference, one precondition that I had set at the outset of the project had not been met. The management and doctors of the outpatient clinic had committed themselves to a zero-growth policy as long as the problems on the ward were not solved. Despite this precondition, there still was an 8 percent increase in the number of new patients over the year, which was one of the main reasons why creating calm at the outpatient clinic proved to be an elusive mission. Freed-up time was easily and rapidly filled. Despite my pointing out that the number of patients had increased during the course of the project, medical specialists could not resist attracting new patients, especially when they wanted to participate in newly initiated studies. When I discussed the increase in the number of new patients with Robert Majoor, one of the leading hematologists, he said, with a not-so-innocent smile, "But that's good, isn't it?" The aim of creating a more livable workplace for doctors' assistants and nurses working extremely hard for a substantially lower salary than their medically trained colleagues turned out to be of secondary importance when weighed against the academic and professional ambitions of this doctor and his colleagues. Despite attempts to make zero growth an immutable aim through quantification (Latour 1987), accepting an increase in production was, for financial and academic reasons, hard to resist. At this stage, it proved impossible for me to re-articulate the issue of the increase of production as a *problem* for the ward. However, some doctors' assistants certainly let me know that the final result of the project was not quite what they had hoped for.

Interventions in Pathways and in Social Studies of Standards

At the outset of this chapter I proposed to explore how experimental social-science research on standardizing health care practices might be interesting for fostering a processual practice of pathwaying based on the notion of situated standardization. This notion proves useful for bypassing the universal/individual dichotomy that runs through many debates and practices of standardization in health care and in other fields. This opposition is particularly unfruitful for overcoming what Martha Lampland and Susan Leigh Star have called "the tyranny of structurelessness" and "the fallacy of one size fits all" (2009, p. v). But rather than proposing that the way out of this dichotomy is to take an "in between" position by standardizing on the niche level of social groups, situated standardization connects standards to specific issues that are sociologically unpacked. Standards then are not a way to overcome a knowledge-practice gap but a way to experimentally reconfigure such gaps. This changes standards from starting points that must be constructed and then implemented in medical practice into standards that Stefan Timmermans and Aaron Mauck call a "rallying point in a comprehensive organizational process of change" (2005, p. 26). Thus, experiments with situated standardization are relevant to pathway development in health care and to furthering sociological debates on standardization.

Situated standardization makes it possible to focus on actual changes in medical practice brought about by standardization and on the perceivable renegotiations of orders and autonomies that come with the standards. This may change the value of pathways from "Taylorist devices for standardizing care and treating each individual in precisely the same way" to "means of affording individualistic treatment, while simultaneously creating organizational efficiency by 'Tayloring' the organisation to the patient (rather than the other way round)" (Pinder et al. 2005, pp. 774–775). This turns the aim of pathways from EBM implementation techniques into processual learning devices for inter-professional quality improvement. As a result of this shift, the pathway is less important than "pathwaying," which opens up new space for doing "politics through standardization" (Timmermans and Berg 2003, p. 216). I would like to propose this form of pathwaying as a practice of situating standardization in specific issues that follow from the analysis of the complexity of a care practice.

Furthermore, there are striking similarities between the value of a processual understanding of pathwaying and the value of developing a situated understanding of the normativity of social-science interventions. Both approaches pre-empt privileging aggregated knowledge—whether normative or clinical—over the complexities of practice. Instead, they situate standardization and normativity in the specificity of the issues that are sociologically unpacked. Both approaches thereby try to avoid the situation in which "the good" is defined outside of the practices to which they are to relate and then have to be "implemented" in. Therefore, both situated standardization and situated intervention can be seen to follow the strategy I call "preventing implementation." I will return to these similarities in the conclusion, but now let me turn to the consequences of situated standardization for what is often seen as its counterpart: patient-centered care.

3   Situated Standardization and Patient-Centered Care

11:00 a.m.

It is a morning in May at the hematology/oncology outpatient clinic and treatment center. I am witnessing what will become a common feature at this hour in the treatment center. Patients waiting for chemotherapy fill the chairs, and many other patients are still waiting for a consult with their hematologist or their oncologist.

At the reception desk, where patients' appointments are scheduled, I find Mrs. and Mr. Walsem waiting. The patient, Mrs. Walsem, lives in the south of the Netherlands and must travel about 200 kilometers to obtain the specialized hematological treatment she needs.

Accompanied by her husband, she has just seen Dr. Van Oost, a junior doctor in training. At the end of the consult, he gave Mrs. Walsem an order sheet, on which he had ticked boxes indicating that she needs a radiology scan and a bone marrow test. The couple took the sheet with them when they returned to reception. Now it is their turn. Fadila, a physician's assistant, is scheduling the required diagnostics. She tries to call a secretary in the radiology department, but all the lines are busy. This is not unusual; radiology is extremely overburdened. Fadila is put on hold. After half an hour, she manages to get through. While she was on hold, she couldn't make appointments. Patient records have piled up. Patients whose consultations have been completed have come back to the reception desk to make follow-up appointments. Some stand in line; others have taken seats near the counter.

Jane, one of Fadila's colleagues, says to me "Of course we could opt to send patients home, and call them back later for their appointments, but then you'd shift the work to after two in the afternoon." I gather that the assistants do not consider that a real option, as other patients will be lining up for new consultations by then.

11:30 a.m.

Mrs. Walsem hears that her radiology scan is scheduled for 8:30 a.m. in a few weeks' time. Mr. Walsem does virtually all the talking, since his wife is very tired. He complains that 8.30 is too early for a patient who must make a three-hour journey to get to the hospital, especially in rush-hour traffic. Besides that, he is unhappy that the bone marrow test is planned for the day before, also at 8:30 a.m.

"But the radiology scan you need is always at 8:30 a.m.," Fadila responds. "There's no changing that. I worked half an hour to get that appointment, and anyway radiology doesn't have time for you the day before." The patient and her husband leave, clearly taken aback, but soon return to the counter. Meanwhile the line has grown longer, and Fadila is helping the next person. Two elderly people come up to complain that they are still waiting when they would like to go home. They are completely worn out. "If there's no time in radiology the day before," Mr. Walsem says insistently to Fadila, "can't we just change the bone marrow test?" Fadila does so, unwillingly.

When the Walsems have gone, Fadila says "It's so annoying, you know. I'm trying to get rid of this pile of patient records, and then you get a patient like this, constantly wanting something else!"

After a while, Mrs. and Mr. Walsem come back yet again. They have called their own internist at their local hospital, and he has told them that they need not go to the university hospital for the radiology scan. It can be done in their local hospital and be sent to the university hospital for further analysis. Mr. Walsem says that they have now made an appointment in their regional hospital. Fadila is helping another patient, and her colleague takes over the Walsems. But Fadila has to intervene anyway to explain the details of what has just taken place. Now the patient Fadila had been helping gets angry with Mrs. Walsem: "Well, I'm standing here waiting, and you just jump the line!" Her husband tries to calm her down.

12:08 p.m.

Dr. Van Oost tells Fadila in passing that Mrs. Walsem needs to get cytogenesis after all, and that Fadila will have to make an appointment for it. She schedules it for the day following the existing appointment for the bone marrow test, and informs Mrs. Walsem, who is still waiting near the counter. Mr. Walsem asks Fadila to change the appointment to the same day as the bone marrow test, and she does so. That involves rescheduling the appointment with the radiology department. It doesn't take half an hour this time, but it does take a long time.

When all the patients are gone, and all the appointments have been made, Dr. Van Oost comes up to the counter after his surgery hours. He asks Fadila how Mrs.

Walsem's appointments were arranged. When he hears the times, he says "Well, actually I won't be there for the bone marrow appointment, because I'm taking a course that day."

Tensions and Alliances Between Standardization and Patient-Centeredness

Situations such as the one described above are, unfortunately, common in outpatient clinics throughout the Western world. When I presented this observation to students on a course on managing changes in health care, one health care manager humorously remarked that this way of organizing treatment is "probably the only thing that is properly standardized in Dutch hospital care." As I noted in the preceding chapter, situated standardization can contribute to improvement of such health care practices in various ways. In this chapter, I address the question "How does such improvement relate to the notion of patient-centered care?"

Since the early 1950s, standardization and patient-centered care have been contrasted strongly in the literature of medical sociology.[1] Standardization has been conceptualized as an ally of the "biomedical model" of medicine, which sociologists criticize for its reductionism and which they contrast with patient-centered ways of delivering care.[2] The aim of the pathwaying experiments in this hospital, however, was to change the organization of care from its focus on managing hospital units to improving patient trajectories by developing standardized care pathways that aim at the pragmatic commensurability of standardization and patient-centeredness. In this chapter I focus on the question of how the concepts of "standardized care trajectories" and "patient-centered care" were related in this setting. How was the dichotomy between standardization and patient-centeredness refigured? What kinds of patient-centered care were enacted through the development of standardized care trajectories? What kinds of standardization matched what forms of patient-centered care? To address these questions, I first explore common conceptualizations and practices of "patient-centeredness" and show how these relate to notions of pathway development.

Dissecting Patient-Centeredness

The opposition between patient-centeredness and standardization has been reinvigorated through the rise of evidence-based medicine. In the literature of medical sociology, patient-centered medicine is increasingly advocated as a response to the proliferation of EBM (Benzing 2000; May et al. 2006; Mead and Bower 2000). In such studies, the limitations of EBM are directly contrasted with patient-centered medicine (PCM), which is said to include "three dimensions of personal care: physical, psychological and social" (Gray 2005, p. 66). Proponents of this dichotomy claim that in "the conventional way of doing medicine, often labeled the 'biomedical model' ... the patient's illness is reduced to a set of signs and symptoms which are investigated and interpreted within a positivist biomedical framework" (Mead and Bower 2000, p. 1088). In contrast, PCM requires a "biopsychosocial perspective" (Scambler 2008, p. 57), which implies a "willingness to become involved in the full range of difficulties patients bring to their doctors, and not just their biomedical problems" (Stewart et al. 1995).[3] This discussion introduces the "patient-centered doctor" (Mead and Bower 2000, p. 1088), who makes all other doctors seem like awkward medical professionals. Patient-centeredness thereby mainly entails a *professional attitude* of seeing patients holistically rather than biomedically. This is what I would like to call the *professional* definition of patient-centeredness.

A second definition of patient-centeredness focuses on a relocation of agency from medical professionals to patients themselves and deals with the direct involvement of patients in the organization and delivery of their care. The US Institute for Healthcare Improvement (IHI) adopted as a motto "Nothing about me without me," which points to patient-centeredness as an attitude that *patients* have to embrace through the political route of direct participation in health care improvement. This second mode is what I would like to call the *participatory* definition of patient-centeredness. In both of these definitions, patient-centered care is mainly about being a "good" "patient-as-person" or "doctor-as-person" (Mead and Bower 2000, pp. 1088–1091), the former requiring a shift by professionals to a holistic perspective on patienthood and the latter conceptualized (similar to the way participatory democrats conceptualize "good" citizenship) as direct involvement in political processes that affect people's lives.

One of the major limitations of these conceptualizations is that they locate solutions for realizing patient-centered care in individuals, and therefore they display little sensitivity for the organizational setting in which these actors relate to one another. Organizational arrangements can merely restrict the professional focus on the wholeness of patients or the democratic purchase for patients to shape the world they inhabit. This polarized discussion is a variation on the dichotomy, which we encountered in the preceding chapter, between the universal and the individualized. Once again EBM is criticized for its homogenizing tendencies, while patient-centered care is presented as taking into account the whole range of issues that matter to the individual patient. Standardization initiatives are held responsible for creating "assembly-line medicine" that, according to George Ritzer (1992, p. 43), will ultimately lead to the "dehumanization and depersonalization of medical practice." Standardizing health care practices thus seems inherently opposed to these definitions of patient-centeredness.

This organization of a particular problem space in which a panacea is diametrically opposed to sociological critique, leaving a highly limited range of options for sociologists to position themselves, is attributable to what Sonja Jerak-Zuiderent calls "the sticky tendencies to get pinned down in either critical or improvement narratives" (2013, p. 158). To resist such tendencies, Jerak-Zuiderent, drawing on the work of Helen Verran and Marilyn Strathern, suggests that it may be worthwhile to pause at the empirical moments that do not fit such narrative orderings. Those moments tend to produce what Helen Verran (2001) calls "disconcertment." They often get left out of analyses precisely because they do not fit dominant narrative orderings. Verran suggests that instead these moments "must be privileged and nurtured, valued and expanded upon." "As a storyteller (a theorist)," she continues, "I treasure these moments. I do not want to explain them away. They are the first clue in my struggle to do useful critique." (ibid., p. 5) Expanding on this suggestion, Jerak-Zuiderent writes:

Such disconcertment, as argued by Marilyn Strathern, is an important entry point for the 'decomposition' of stories, which she describes as "taking apart an image to see/ make visible what inside it contains" (1992, p. 245). This does not equal 'debunking' by an outside perspective, but rather a process in which "the elicitor/witness is in a crucial sense the "creator" of the image, and his/her presence [is] thus necessary to its appearance" (ibid.). This very move positions me, as an analyst, in the midst of the scene as a "witness to [my] own efforts of elucidation" (ibid.). It demands an analytical sensitivity to how these very efforts interweave with the world I research and the stories I tell." (in press)

In this chapter, I follow suggestions that state that "interruptions, small and large are what we, as theorists, must learn to value and use" (Verran 2001, p. 5) and that propose that we analyze the interferences in our narratives for their potential to "slow down this plot" (Jerak-Zuiderent, in press) of predictable solutions and their oppositions and critique. I do so by decomposing some events at the clinic that at first sight seemed to constitute a rather sticky, if not caricature-like, narrative on standardization and patient-centeredness as antonyms. Upon closer analysis, however, it turned out that even when it sometimes precluded professionally situated assessments or patients' democratic autonomy, standardization was able to contribute to a more *organizational* definition of patient-centeredness. To decompose the sticky narratives on standardization and patient-centeredness, let me now turn to analyzing the doctors I encountered who seemed to perfectly match the images of the "biomedical doctor" and the "patient-centered doctor." At first it seemed unlikely that I would find a doctor whose practice could even remotely be described as "interrupting the patient's 'voice of the lifeworld' with response-constraining questions, [while] the doctor's 'voice of medicine' effectively strips away the personal meaning of the illness" (Mead and Bower 2000, p. 1089). Yet it seemed as if I had found exactly such a doctor at the hematology/oncology outpatient clinic.

Biomedical Doctoring? If "Dexamethasone" Is the Right Answer

In chapter 2 we came across the strong variation in the number of patients different oncologists were seeing during surgery. (See table 2.1.) The differences were directly related to the varying work routines of different physicians. During a surgery I observed, Dr. Fuchs had 17 patients booked in 12 slots. Many patients had been booked between his regular slots, which sometimes reduced the 20 minutes per follow-up visit that was the norm for this clinic to about five minutes. In these visits, he welcomed the patients, went through a checklist for their trial with them, physically examined them, for which some had to undress, and sometimes gave practical advice about ways of dealing with the consequences of treatment. He would, for example, advise a patient who was having trouble swallowing because of the treatment for his esophagus carcinoma to adjust his eating habits: "Just eat dry toast instead of fresh bread. It's like when you're going fishing and you make a sticky ball of fresh bread. Or like an hourglass: the sand runs through as long as it's dry, but if you add water, it clogs right away."

During the consultations, Dr. Fuchs was busily looking for lab results in the hospital information system, filling out forms, writing in the patient record. He barely looked at the patients. When he showed the way to a patient who had come to the treatment center for the first time, he walked so fast that the patient and his wife headed off in the wrong direction because they had lost sight of him. He had to go after them and call them back.

Patients who had been undergoing treatment by Dr. Fuchs for some time seemed accustomed to such quick, efficient, biomedical encounters. Once the doctor asked "Do you need anything?" and the patient answered "Dexamethasone," obviously thinking that a request for cancer medication was the right answer, and that "a talk about problems at home due to treatment stress" or "more time to think before starting the next course of treatment" would be inappropriate. Often there seemed to be very little space for "the voice of the lifeworlds" that patients inhabit and that advocates of patient-centered care try to move to center stage. The vignette that follows is illustrative.

Mr. Vukovic is a Croatian who has almost no voice, probably as a result of treatment for carcinoma of the esophagus. His wife does all the talking. Mr. Vukovic wheezes that he needs more time before his next course of treatment starts. Mrs. Vukovic says that she went to Croatia for three weeks to let herself be spoiled by her family in her own house, but she came back earlier, because she had noticed that her husband was not doing at all well.

"What's the problem?" asks Dr. Fuchs.

Mrs. Vukovic replies "Mentally, he's just not doing well. He could prepare himself for the previous courses of chemotherapy, and then it works out, but now it's totally unexpected, and he just can't deal with it."

"Yes, but of course we didn't plan it like that," says Dr. Fuchs. "He just responded well and so we said, well, let's go on right away."

I'm wondering how "we" decided this when Mrs. Vukovic says "But he's having such a hard time. I can just tell. And he can't sleep at night at all, he's very afraid. Then I have to hold his hand really tight and stroke his head. And he says 'But then the doctor will be angry if I don't want to go on.' So I say 'The doctor won't get mad, he can't.' Can you? And he [Mr. Vukovic] is so very worried about his feet. He still has this strange sensation there. And he's always outside, except when he's asleep. But soon he'll have to stay inside: he just can't do that! I can tell: I've been looking at this man for 35 years, sad to say." She says it lovingly, clutching her husband's arm.

Dr. Fuchs asks about the tingling sensation in Mr. Vukovic's feet and fingers. Saying that he has already explained this, once again the doctor points out that the sensation is due to damage to the fine nerves. It comes from the chemotherapy and is a side effect that generally disappears, but sometimes stays.

"But if my husband has to go on living like a pathetic little man, that's no good either!" Mrs. Vukovic says.

"Yes, quality of life matters too," Dr. Fuchs agrees.

"He's getting so forgetful. He forgets his keys and everything. He never used to do that!"

"Well, that can't be due to the treatment," Dr. Fuchs says. He then suggests that Mr. Vukovic gets a one-week postponement for starting the next chemotherapy, also because his current blood values don't allow a new course of treatment right away. But he also says that he can't afford to wait another two months just because Mr. Vukovic is insecure. "Then I wouldn't have a clue what I'm doing anymore."

I find the consult confrontational. There is so little space for the reasonable fears, doubts, and worries of Mr. and Mrs. Vukovic. And how can Dr. Fuchs be so sure that the forgetfulness is not due to the treatment—if only in a psychosomatic sense, perhaps?

Dr. Fuchs comes back from the counter, where he went to hand over the order sheets and pick up his next patients. He walks faster than his next patients, and before they enter he says to me about the Vukovices "They're a pretty bizarre couple. He used to booze it up and throw his weight around, act the big leader. Now she takes charge a bit. I've noticed because they've been seeing me since ... [he looks in the electronic record] 1998."

At first sight it seemed that I had identified a doctor of the sort described in the literature on patient-centeredness as representing the "biomedical model." However, it would have been too easy to caricature this doctor without finding out what he knows about the "life-world" of his patients. It turned out that there was more to his knowledge of his patients than my initial observation of the clinic revealed. And because of his efficiency in dealing with patients, he was able to see many patients in a short time— which meant that in spite of high demand on the surgery hours, the time of admission to the clinic had stayed within a week. Did his unholistic approach, which nonetheless made possible short admission times for severely ill patients, merely contradict patient-centeredness?

Patient-Centered Professionals? The Doctor as Travel Agent

When I tried to identify a "patient-centered doctor" in this clinic, once again I did not have to look long. Table 2.1 showed that some doctors seemed to spend far more time on their patients than Dr. Fuchs did, and indeed Dr. Busse took all the time her patients required—up to 45 minutes or even more for a consultation planned to last for 20 minutes (and one that Dr. Fuchs would complete in about five minutes). Observing Dr. Busse's clinic was a very different experience. She fully displayed the "willingness to become involved in the full range of difficulties patients bring to their doctors, and not just their biomedical problems" that the PCM approach prescribes, and she seemed a true "doctor-as-person" seeing "patients-as-people." Dr. Busse was willing to discuss any problem that a patient encountered and defined nothing as beyond her scope.

During the long consult Dr. Busse and Mrs. Marconi discuss when exactly to start the next course of chemotherapy. Mrs. Marconi says that her main problem is not deciding when to start the course, but deciding how to deal with the uncertainty of the treatment for her ovary carcinoma: "I know we're trying hard, but I also know that chances are that my days are numbered. I would really like to visit my daughter, who's living in Florida, because, you know, it may be the last time. But if I book my flight now, and my blood values are low, I'll have to postpone my course and can't catch my flight."

"In that case," Dr. Busse replies, "booking a last-minute flight is probably for the best. There are some really good websites for last-minute bookings, and that way you don't have to worry about booking ahead." She goes on to explain which websites offer such vacations at best rates, and that Mrs. Marconi can also book an entire last-minute vacation, including accommodations, but can use only the flight and stay with her daughter.

Although Dr. Busse seemed to be giving her patients a remarkable degree of care, they had to spend a long time in the waiting room before she had time for them. Often patients who were scheduled later in the morning, or in the afternoon, called in advance to hear how far behind schedule Dr. Busse was running so they could adjust their time of arrival accordingly. Her "patient-centered" approach also meant that the assistants either couldn't take lunch breaks or had to do extra work in the afternoon to deal with work that had piled up in the morning. If the doctor had an afternoon clinic, they could not go home on time, or they would have to leave a pile of records for patients needing appointments for the morning crew to deal with.

And the problem seemed more substantial than just the extra-long waits for patients and delayed lunch breaks for staff. At the start of the project, Dr. Busse declined my invitation for an interview, saying that she didn't have time for it and that she preferred to spend her precious time on patient care. When I mentioned that to Dr. Fuchs, who was also the medical manager of the oncology unit, he was very annoyed. He summoned a secretary to make an appointment for my interview with Dr. Busse, and the interview was scheduled for a few days later.

As I had expected, Dr. Busse was late for the interview, but at least she showed up. However, her first sentences made it apparent that she was not going to cooperate willingly. As I was explaining the project and the aim of improving the organization of care on the hematology/oncology ward, she interrupted me. Referring to a slogan the hospital had begun using, she snapped "And 'putting patients center stage,' where does that fit in?" The exchange continued as follows:

TZJ: You miss that?

Dr. Busse: I don't know, I don't see it.

TZJ: What do you mean, you don't see it?

Dr. Busse: Well, where do you see it?

TZJ: Well you should start seeing it in this project when patients who now have to wait a long time to arrange their diagnostic trajectory will be helped far more smoothly.

Rather than let me take on the role of interviewer and make her do the talking, Dr. Busse took over the interview and forced me to justify my good intentions. However, she was obviously not convinced, and soon she interrupted again. Pointing at the recording device, she said "One more thing: What will happen to the recording? Who has access to it?" Her suspicion was not without grounds. Later I became aware that her position within the department had been a subject of considerable debate. Complaints from her colleagues about her clinics always running late had reached the department chair. After many unfruitful and sometimes hostile discussions about the need to reduce the time she spent per patient, they chose an alternative route to bring her surgery back under control. Ward management restricted the number of patients she was allowed to see. She was given a strict maximum of seven patients per clinic, while others had twelve slots and were actually seeing up to eighteen patients in four hours. As Dr. Busse's slots quickly filled up, patients who did not fit her schedule were booked with her colleagues instead. According to Dr. Busse, this was highly inefficient:

We must be able to treat our patients properly, our own patients, and not ad hoc from one to the next doctor. That makes you lose grip and leads to things going wrong, which is not in the best interest of patients or in our own. It seems like you're being relieved but it gives twice as much work, because this other doctor sees the patient once in between other things; he doesn't have the story or the policy in his head. And then sometimes things are not done properly, or they miss certain things. It's just not in the interest of the chemotherapy course. Afterwards all the things that must be arranged land on my desk, all the phone calls about things that are not correct. Ultimately, if you take just a bit more time in the surgery hour, you would be finished so much earlier.

As I found out later, Dr. Busse had not kept her frustration to herself. When patient numbers were limited for her clinics, patients quickly noticed a huge change in doctoring style. They were not accustomed to indicating their need for medication when asked if they needed anything, as the patients of Dr. Fuchs were, and they were shocked by the sudden change. If Dr. Busse met a patient in the corridors and the patient expressed concern, she urged the patient to file a complaint with the department chair about the new policy and the reduced quality of care. As formal complaints require careful attention, answering all the letters of complaint eventually became too much of a burden for Hans van Barneveld, the head of the department (a highly renowned, busy professor), and he let go of his demands. I didn't find out about this until later, though. During the interview with Dr. Busse, I discussed another way of dealing with the problem of her surgery hours. I proposed that she allow a nurse-practitioner to take over substantial parts of the treatment and that she improve her collaboration with the nurse-practitioner and with other professional colleagues by resuming a weekly oncology meeting. Dr. Busse responded as follows:

Well, but of course, it is … we can do without a doctor. I see people from community hospitals who tell me they saw a doctor at the start and the end of the chemotherapy but not during. So yes, it's possible, I guess, it could work out fine with all these nurse-practitioners. But I'm used to intervening a bit and it's easy enough to steer them away from little complaints. That's why I see people briefly [before each dose of chemotherapy]. An oncology meeting doesn't cover everything and I think it shouldn't; it would only take more time. I thought we were working on solutions?! To improve things?!

Later it became clear that there was more to Dr. Busse's criticism than the issue of inefficiency introduced by treating patients with a team of professionals. One day I ran into a nurse named Ellen just as she was leaving the day care treatment center. She was trying to escape the treatment center quickly, and she was visibly distressed. I went with her and asked what was wrong. She replied "I just can't take Dr. Busse's stress schemes anymore! We're driving these patients to death!"

Ellen explained that the rigid trial protocols also include standards for "stress schemes" prescribing how to act when patients have adverse reactions to their chemotherapy, and that break periods of certain durations are specified. For example, patients must take 30-minute breaks before they can have a second attempt at taking the course. But such breaks cannot be given perpetually. Trial protocols clearly indicate after how many adverse reactions a patient must stop the course of chemotherapy. Obviously this can be a dramatic decision in tertiary oncology care, as it can easily mean that the only form of treatment left is palliative care. However, Dr. Busse employed her own stress schemes in instances when a patient had more reactions than the trial allowed. She introduced additional 30-minute breaks, after which she re-started the course even if the patient's adverse reactions had crossed the limit set by the protocol.

Ellen had just administered such a course to a patient who was no longer able to bear the treatment. Ellen criticized Dr. Busse for overruling the biomedical limits set to the treatment. According to Ellen, adjusting stress schemes stopped patients from focusing on the end of their life, for which they first needed to accept that there was no longer the chance of a cure. As it turned out, Dr. Busse's complete focus on patients' individual wishes reversed the situation so that they were *under her complete control*. The patient-centered repertoire provided unprecedented space for a medicalization of her patients that went much further than biomedical standard treatment protocols would ever permit.

The way Dr. Busse reacted to proposals for any kind of multi-professional cooperation—e.g., a weekly oncology meeting, letting colleagues see her patients, and (later) introducing nurse-practitioners—were not merely attempts to prevent the segmentation of holistic care, but were endeavors to prevent any form of inter-professional accountability of the care she delivered. Focusing primarily on patient-centered care situated *in the interpersonal encounter* between a patient and a doctor providing holistic care meant that other possible issues in delivering highly complex patient-centered care were easily overlooked. Any sentimental attachment to understanding PCM as a matter of the attitude of professionals toward their patients would easily lead to telling the story of Dr. Busse in terms of the sticky narrative that opposes patient-centeredness with standardization. It would have been easy to tell a story about the attempts of patient-centered doctors to resist managerial attempts at standardizing health care work. It could easily be positioned in a narrative about professionalism's being challenged by managerialism, with a pinch of neoliberalism and a pinch of marketization as recognizable tasty ingredients. But even when I found out that Dr. Busse was unwilling to let me interview her about her work and possible improvements she could envision, I felt disconcerted, and that made me want to unpack the story on patient-centeredness a little further. Although I was certainly sympathetic to her approach to her patients, I started to get the feeling that what on first sight looked sympathetic and patient-centered might in practice turn out to be quite coercive (cf. Silverman 1987). As decomposing the event of patient-centered doctoring by Dr. Busse showed, the risk that patient-centered care may give doctors unprecedented power tells quite a different story about the relationship between patient-centered care and standardization, and the dark side of resisting standardization is not attended to sufficiently in the literature of medical sociology.

Participatory Patient-Centeredness? Nothing About Me Without Me

Patient involvement was not mentioned in the research design for the improvement project at the hematology/oncology outpatient clinic. One reason was that the doctors responded skeptically to the idea during our discussions about setting up the research. They preferred to see my time dedicated to analyzing data from the hospital information system and problems on the ward. The skepticism wasn't attributable to their not valuing patients' opinions. It stemmed partly from doubts about the usefulness of asking patients about their experiences. Physicians mentioned how surprised they were that they still tended to score well on patient-satisfaction questionnaires, even though they felt that they faced substantial organizational problems. I was aware of this problem of high scores for poor organizations, which is well documented in the literature of medical sociology.[4] In previous projects I had also noticed that patients tended to appreciate the enormous efforts professionals made to serve them. Since they are generally not in a position to see how organizational problems could be prevented, patients value the "ad-hocking" that goes on, seeing it as still giving them the best possible care under difficult circumstances. They see these efforts as a sign of the laudable commitment of health care workers rather than a sign of poor organization, which it may very well be. Poor organization can thus easily contribute to high satisfaction rates.

Another reason the doctors put forward for not including patients in the project was that it would require approval by a medical ethics review board, which would delay the project and prevent us from actually addressing the problems we already could articulate. I felt strongly that the doctors used this reason to dismiss the somewhat touchy subject of patient involvement, but it meant it was impossible for me to include patient interviews as part of the initial set-up of the research.

However, patients were included in the project in three ways. First, they were all around us. I observed their interactions with personnel at the clinic on my participant observation days. They became accustomed to seeing me around, and they approached me freely to share their experiences. Second, I happened to get informally acquainted with a patient who had been treated on the ward for more than ten years. Interestingly, this veteran patient was an organizational advisor for a large Dutch consultancy firm, which put him in an excellent position to think with me about how to prevent organizational problems. We had several extensive meetings to discuss proposed changes, and I spoke freely with this "expert patient" in private. He was willing and able to give valuable input on organizational matters from his perspective as a patient, and his experience with the management of change far exceeded mine. Third, during a later stage of the project the doctors and I developed a brief questionnaire for patients in the treatment center that contained questions about their treatment experiences. It included questions such as "Have you had any adverse reaction that you were not told would be a risk of the treatment? If so, what was your reaction?" We used this questionnaire to assess the accuracy of the information patients received about their treatment.

I could tell from patients' identification numbers what treatments they had received. When I discussed the matches with hematologists and oncologists, we found that patients were often surprised by common reactions that should have been routinely explained during the visit prior to commencing treatment. We were unable to assess whether this indicated that patients had not been informed properly or whether it indicated that they had forgotten being informed because they had heard too much information at once. No matter the reason, we interpreted the responses as valid for patients' experiences at the treatment center. The responses also confirmed the failure to inform patients directly before starting their chemotherapy, as discussed in chapter 2. A question worth exploring is whether clandestine patient participation, rather than letting patients take the lead in health care improvement, makes this study problematic in terms of patient-centeredness, as the participatory definition would suggest. Surely the way patient-centeredness was positioned in this project did not comply with "Nothing About Me Without Me," the slogan used by the Institute for Healthcare Improvement.

From a participatory standpoint on the matter of patient-centeredness, the fact that patients began writing letters of complaint to the department chair about changes in the arrangement of their care could easily be seen as a good step in the direction of patient empowerment. However, that extreme case of patient-centeredness equally shows that defining patient-centeredness as patient involvement not only limits professionals in their attempts to clinically "strip away the personal meaning of the illness," as Mead and Bower would have it, but also sometimes excessively empowers care professionals to manipulate patients. This disconcerting moment during my research does thereby point to some important tensions in the participatory approach to patient-centeredness. One tension pointed out by critics of participative democracy is that power relations at play in such settings are often obscured by the focus on participative rhetoric (Markussen 1996). In a health care setting that tries to improve its patient-centeredness, "playing the patient card" is a powerful strategy, especially when the patients are highly controlled by individual medical professionals.

A second problem is that participatory definitions of patient-centeredness assume that patients want to be involved, to be fully informed, and to be the ones making the choices about the care they are receiving. Such assumptions about the involvement of patients have proved highly problematic in medical research. Steve Epstein (2007, chapter 9) describes the emergence of hordes of "recruitmentologists" striving to meet inclusion criteria for patients in clinical trials. Though no such industry has sprung up for quality-improvement initiatives yet, agents of quality improvement face similar problems in finding patients willing to participate, which points to the fact that participatory patient-centeredness may require a fair amount of non-patient initiated action before patients are included in the design of their own care.[5] A deliberately democratic view of patienthood therefore raises questions about the desirability of patients' being enacted as inherently having a "perspective" (Pols 2005). It raises further questions about whether patients not only should be able to *choose* their care but also should *bear responsibility for* any *consequences* they may suffer as a result of their active participation (Mol 2008). Participatory approaches problematize the patients' right to depend on the expertise of care providers and delegate part of the burden of responsibility to patients. The philosopher of technology Hans Harbers voices these problems of participatory approaches as follows:

In emphasizing the formal rights to participate, for example, [a participatory approach] tends to disregard substantial differences—differences in power as well as differences in expertise. Or, to mention one more criticism, the theory of deliberative democracy is rather optimistic about the will of both experts and laymen to learn and participate. As if everybody wants to deliberate about everything all the time. According to the normative commitments of deliberative democracy, this should in fact be assumed as a moral responsibility by citizens. But that denies the human right on political laziness—a right so elegantly accounted for in systems of *indirect, representational* democracy, delegating our political duties to elected political professionals for a couple of years (2005b, p. 266).

Such critiques[6] of the model of participatory or "strong" democracy should make us aware of the conceptual implications for participatory notions of patient-centeredness. They imply that, rather than enact patient-centeredness as either a quality that individual doctors should develop or a procedural approach to including patients in redesigning care, it is worthwhile to consider how standardization may *not* be antithetical to a more organizational approach to patient-centeredness.

Pathwaying and Patient-Centeredness as Outcomes

In chapter 2 we saw how the organization of care at the hematology/oncology outpatient clinic was changed substantially by rigorously preparing for intake consults, improving the planning of diagnostics by creating slots in the radiology department, and referring much of the follow-up back to general hospitals. These were not merely organizational interventions to improve the management of the clinic; they were materializations of care that is organized around the trajectories of patients and the work of professionals. What organizational patient-centeredness entailed in practice was, however, always the outcome of an experimental process of situated-intervention research. This differs from the other definitions of patient-centeredness in an important way. Whereas the professional definition requires a change of attitude by doctors, and the participatory definition a procedural approach to placing patients in the lead, an organizational approach entails empirically testing what patient-centeredness may mean when it is situated in the complexity of a specific care practice. What organizational patient-centered care is, therefore, can be learned only if we, in Hacking's words (1983, p. 149), "'twist the lion's tail'—that is, manipulate our world in order to learn its secrets." Francis Bacon's metaphor for producing uncontentiously realist knowledge about phenomena is particularly appropriate. "Twisting the lion's tail" implies a warning that a tuition fee may be charged when actors roar—especially in response to looming sentimentality about a certain effort to make care patient-centered.

From the start of this project, I had been quite sympathetic to the idea of introducing nurse-practitioners into the organization of cancer treatment. I recognized there was substantial controversy about the idea among oncologists, but I saw this as due mainly to professional conservatism and the relatively low professional status of nurses in the Dutch health care system. Introducing nurse-practitioners into the organization of oncological treatment seemed to make sense for several reasons

First, as was discussed in the preceding chapter, space in surgery hours could be freed up for hematologists through various efficiency gains, but inefficiencies in for example return visits and clogged surgery hours due to much late follow-up were less of a problem for oncologists. In most cases, cancer treatment or follow-up could not be referred back to general hospitals, because oncologists had no dependable system in place for ensuring the reliability of trial data, as was the case for hematology care. Setting up collaborative system with other hospitals would take far longer than the project allowed, so we needed alternative ways to create space in overcrowded clinics.

Second, other university hospitals were showing impressive results from the introduction of nurse-practitioners in their outpatient clinics. Several members of the oncology working group attended a presentation at another Dutch university hospital in which a nurse-practitioner spoke about the substantial reduction of the patient return rate, enthusiastic patients, and a level of professional autonomy of qualified nurses that was almost becoming problematic now that the oncologists barely showed their faces on the ward, content to leave treatment under the supervision of these "new professionals." General hospitals were increasingly working with nurse-practitioners, and were happy to share their experiences by giving a presentation about these developments at the university hospital. This was a thorn in the flesh of some oncologists and hematologists, who were very annoyed that the nurses had invited a nurse-practitioner from a general hospital to give a presentation at their ward, when the university hospital was supposed to be leading the developments. Though this embarrassment caused some tension, at least it demonstrated that the ward would fall behind the others if it did not join the development of introducing nurse-practitioners.

Third, and perhaps most important, I was inspired by studies that showed how the work of nurses often has a particular kind of invisibility that could be made a more explicit part of care on the ward by introducing new professional roles. The work of nurses often is invisible, though not in the sense that it cannot be observed. "If one looked," Star and Strauss wrote (1999, p. 20), "one could literally see the work being done—but the taken-for-granted status means that it is functionally invisible." Though it has been shown that undoing such functional invisibility risks making nursing work deal with more surveillance and heaps of cumbersome paperwork (Wagner 1993), as well as risking "the eradication of discretion from skilled workers" (Star and Strauss 1999, pp. 20–21), I was optimistic that, in combination with the increased professional status that nurse-practitioners would acquire, this change would mainly contribute to making care more patient-centered.

In spite of problems that had arisen from earlier attempts to change the surgery hours on this ward, I managed to convince some of the oncologists, including Otto Reimers, the professor of oncology overseeing the project, that introducing a nurse-practitioner could reduce the oncologists' return rate and the time they needed to spend on each patient. Large portions of treatment could be delegated to the new professional, which hopefully would free up time in regular oncology surgery hours. Yet the initiative for introducing a nurse-practitioner was not much of a success. I spent several sessions with the oncologists drafting a scheme for the nurse-practitioner's tasks in one of the simplest care trajectories: that for testis carcinoma. (See figure 3.1.) There was a clear clinical practice guideline for the treatment of patients with this disease. Most of the care is a medically straightforward late follow-up, which because of the low incidence of the disease is restricted to university hospitals. Therefore, testis carcinoma seemed an ideal case for specifying nurse-practitioners' tasks (the second box in the legend of figure 3.1) and defining the moments when they should contact an oncologist (the first box in the legend of figure 3.1). Clicking on one of the "nurse-practitioner" boxes led to more detailed pages (exemplified

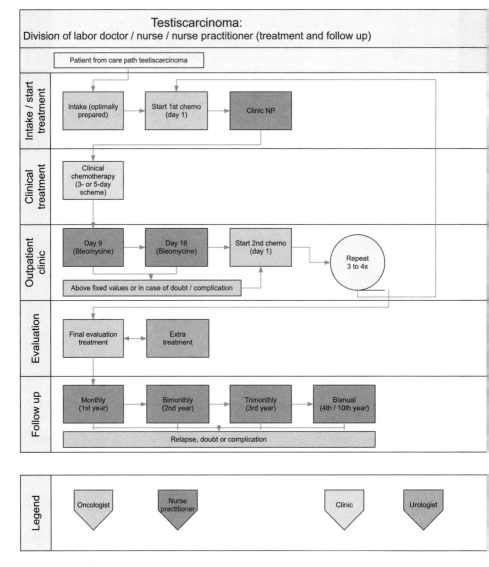

Figure 3.1
Re-delegation of tasks to a nurse-practitioner in the treatment of testis carcinoma.

here by figure 3.2) specifying the extent to which nurse-practitioners could act without contacting an oncologist. The standardization was more about defining the limits of autonomous action than about prescribing detailed actual activities.

After the re-delegation of work was standardized, there was a heated debate between some of the oncology nurses and Dr. Busse. The discussion

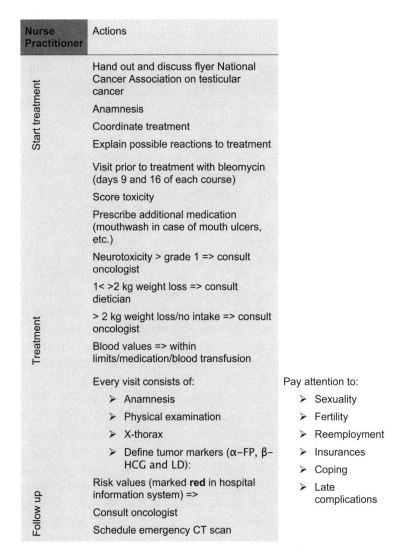

Nurse Practitioner	Actions	
Start treatment	Hand out and discuss flyer National Cancer Association on testicular cancer	
	Anamnesis	
	Coordinate treatment	
	Explain possible reactions to treatment	
Treatment	Visit prior to treatment with bleomycin (days 9 and 16 of each course)	
	Score toxicity	
	Prescribe additional medication (mouthwash in case of mouth ulcers, etc.)	
	Neurotoxicity > grade 1 => consult oncologist	
	1< >2 kg weight loss => consult dietician	
	> 2 kg weight loss/no intake => consult oncologist	
	Blood values => within limits/medication/blood transfusion	
Follow up	Every visit consists of: ➢ Anamnesis ➢ Physical examination ➢ X-thorax ➢ Define tumor markers (α–FP, β–HCG and LD):	Pay attention to: ➢ Sexuality ➢ Fertility ➢ Reemployment ➢ Insurances ➢ Coping ➢ Late complications
	Risk values (marked **red** in hospital information system) =>	
	Consult oncologist	
	Schedule emergency CT scan	

Figure 3.2
Specification of nurse-practitioners' tasks for testis carcinoma.

among the oncologists became further polarized when, during an improvement meeting, Dr. Busse made a remark that was entirely in line with the sociological idea of "biopsychosocial doctoring": "Psychosocial care is an integral part of treatment that can only be done by a doctor. Nurses simply cannot do that." Then Dr. Evers, an oncologist who specialized in the most experimental trials, replied that what they were discussing was nothing but "monkey medicine" (i.e., medical work that even a well-trained ape could do), and all chances of a fruitful conversation were effectively eliminated.

Furthermore, I was beginning to doubt that some of the nurses in this outpatient clinic matched my view of skilled professionals with functionally invisible capabilities, even if they were ready to take up the responsibility of undergoing the advanced training required of a nurse-practitioner. The manager of the nursing staff had begun breathing new life into the practice of holding professionalization sessions on the ward as part of the improvement project. The oncology nurses on this ward did not seem to display the same professional spirit as the highly specialized hemophilia nurses we met in chapter 1, who were committed to learning more about their patients and new forms of treatment by attending conferences and engaging in inter-professional exchanges with other hemophilia nurses throughout the country. Since it was an outpatient clinic and a day care treatment center, many of the oncology nurses valued the fact that they never had to work nights or weekends, which was an important reason why many of them to wanted to work there. The manager of the nursing staff tried to kindle their enthusiasm for learning about new forms of cancer treatment by inviting a speaker from another hospital to talk on this topic. The speaker wanted to go through some of the basics of regular treatment on the ward, then quickly move on to innovative treatment methods, but soon he realized that the basics raised so many questions that the whole session would have to be devoted to things that should have been common knowledge. Later, when the oncologists and hematologists heard about this, they said it confirmed their doubts about the professional skills of their nursing staff. I had managed to secure funding for two nurses to take the training needed to become nurse-practitioners, but I knew that hiring new nurse-practitioners was out of the question. That was when I realized that the delegation of tasks was not going to work. Management at the unit formally declined the proposal to introduce nurse-practitioners, although all realized that it could have contributed to creating calm and organizationally patient-centered care on the ward. This shows that, in exploring the relationship between patient-centeredness and standardization, standards must not be evaluated solely on the basis of what they include but also by what they omit (Bowker and Star 1999).

Yet the net outcome of the experiment was more than just some nice flow charts that did little to create organizational patient-centeredness. Recognizing that it was not feasible to press for more formalized re-delegation of tasks to nurse-practitioners, we decided that the project could still pursue the redistribution of work, but that it should do so more modestly by introducing a simpler nurse-led clinic for oncology patients. All the nurses had become used to this set-up, as it had already proved successful in the development of the hemophilia care center. (See chapter 1.) This clinic was also an attempt to create a much-needed collaborative connection between oncologists and nurses, as now they would have to begin working together and discussing their findings during consults. This strategy proved fruitful about three months after the end of the study. In a meeting on how the situation at the ward could be further improved, nurses and doctors agreed that the former would attend the oncology meetings at which patients were discussed—a move that had been unimaginable just a few months earlier. The oncologists were opening up to the nurses, and during their consults with patients the nurses began to notice that their limited knowledge of care on the ward really was a problem, as patients often were well informed and raised questions the nurses were not always able to answer. This made them eager to learn more, not just to be able to serve patients better but also to avoid the embarrassment of being at a loss for words when patients asked them such questions. Oncologists and oncology nurses also expressed a wish to further explore the possibilities for delegating more administrative and planning-related tasks to nurses. Clearly they had begun to prepare for a more substantial redistribution of work and responsibility. What organizational patient-centeredness entails is, therefore, not a matter of clearly defining the boundaries of professional responsibilities; it is, rather, an outcome of a dynamic process of standardization.

Situated Intervention and Organizational Patient-Centeredness

Rather than situating patient-centered care in the attitude of doctors, or in the procedural involvement of patients, I argue for the advantages of producing patient-centeredness through a process of sociological experiments in the organization of care delivery. First, this makes patient-centeredness specific, located, and (con-)testable. Relocating patient-centered care in sociologically explored issues that one faces in the delivery of care proved crucial for arriving at a substantive definition of patient-centeredness.

Professional or participatory definitions carry stronger preconceived notions about when patient-centeredness is being achieved; in a professional understanding, this is when the doctors' attitude changes, and in a participatory understanding when patients are involved in redesigning their care. An organizational definition of patient-centeredness calls for more specification of how certain organizational standards may contribute to certain aspects of patient-centeredness. Standardizing the organization of care and making it more patient-centered are, therefore, neither inherently opposed nor intrinsically positively related. From this follows the need to specify how standards are in fact relating to patient-centeredness, which may well reduce the risk of extreme marginalization of patients currently taking place under the banner of patient-centeredness. Not only are these other definitions unable to prevent such excesses; they also risk contributing to reproducing sticky narratives about the relationship between standardization and patient-centeredness that obscure, rather than illuminate, such unforeseen dynamics.

Second, this approach also provides the sociology of invisible work with important insights. Though I started with a familiar sociological attachment to the invisible skilled work of marginalized professional groups, much in line with the "underdog" concern that runs widely through sociology, experimenting with the introduction of nurse-practitioners challenged this attachment when I found that, besides invisible *skilled* work, there is substantial invisible *unskilled* work, which made the proposed change of delegating tasks to nurses highly problematic. This points to the importance of making use of disconcerting moments to prevent a sociological attachment to hidden skills from turning into a sentimental attachment that blinds sociologists to hidden *in*abilities of nurses and other marginalized knowledge workers.

I hope to have shown that experiments in situated intervention, with their focus on the dynamic process of the articulation of sociological issues, can refigure how care can be made patient-centered in more substantial and relevant ways. The meaning of this relevance is better specified *in situ* than defined in abstract sentimentality. Moreover, twisting the lion's tail and experiencing how that makes the lion roar provides rich opportunities for the production of sociological knowledge on invisible work and for decomposing "roaring" events.

Let me now turn to the potential of situated intervention for experimenting with the regulatory infrastructure of health care markets.

4   The Qualities of Competition: Reconfiguring Health Care Markets

In 1999 the Atrium Medical Center, a large teaching hospital in the hilly south of the Netherlands, did something that many hospitals were doing at the time: it introduced a "joint care" trajectory for patients receiving hip or knee prostheses. After the development of "total hip" or "total knee" implants in the preceding decades, and with more and more patients receiving such prostheses (Faulkner 2002), the 1990s saw intensified efforts to provide hip-replacement and knee-replacement surgery to several patients on the same day (Schrijvers, Oudendijk, and de Vries 2003). Clustering operations in small groups, typically of five patients, produced a group dynamic that shortened hospital stays. In addition to improving intramural coordination, the Atrium Medical Center reduced the average length of stay of hip-replacement and knee-replacement patients from 18 days to about 6 days—a dramatic improvement in service, with decreased costs for the hospital and reduced discomfort for the patients.

In May of 2005, a nearby clinic at the Maasland Hospital announced that it had developed a new care arrangement, called Healing Hills, that would quickly transfer patients to a nearby luxury hotel—the Chateau St Gerlach (figure 4.1)—after joint-replacement surgery. They could then recover in pleasant surroundings in a facility that brought together "the highest quality of care and the hospitality of Limburg."[1] The hospital developed this arrangement in cooperation with one of the smaller health insurance companies in the region, which was preparing itself for changes in the health insurance market that would take effect in 2006, when the Healthcare Market Regulation Act would be introduced. That act replaced the traditional Dutch system for budgeting the delivery of care by means of a mixed system of mandatory public and voluntary private insurances with a system much in line with the "Obamacare" initiative in the United States: all citizens were obliged to be insured by private insurance companies. Health insurance providers would henceforth have to compete for clients and negotiate with hospitals on the quality and price of the "care products" they offered. In creating an image of its insurance package as combining high-quality clinical care with the typical southern Dutch *savoir vivre*, the insurance company hoped to attract many new customers in a region with an aging population.

The announcement of the care provided by the Maasland Hospital received substantial local press coverage. Although the managers and doctors of the Atrium Medical Center laughed the "innovation" off as "mere window dressing," they also recognized the potential consequences of this stunt for their own facility's image and recognized that something should be done. They were aware that the Atrium Medical Center could not compete with the service levels that the Maasland Hospital was offering, but they figured that, on an economic level, they could become a far more interesting partner for the insurance companies if they could make the goal of their joint care trajectory substantially cheaper delivery of higher-quality medical care. This was particularly interesting because on January 1, 2005, the Netherlands introduced a new financing system for hospital care. Before 2005, funds were barely connected to the actual activities hospitals carried out, since the funding of hospitals was based on availability, capacity, and production. This scheme was replaced with a system of diagnosis-related groups, and prices for common medical procedures became freely

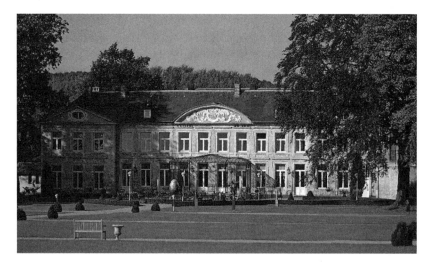

Figure 4.1
Chateau St Gerlach. Courtesy of Chateau St Gerlach.

negotiable between hospitals and insurance companies. Since hip replacements and knee replacements are among the freely negotiable procedures, the management of the Atrium Medical Center saw low price as an important selling point in the upcoming round of negotiations with insurers. With their orthopedic surgeons, management decided to have a close look at their joint-care trajectory and realized that by running an improvement project they could further reduce the length of stay for a total hip replacement to 4½ days and that for a total knee replacement to 3½ days. Hospital management and surgeons also figured they could expand the inclusion criteria for the joint care service so that 80 percent of all patients needing a new hip or knee could be treated this way instead of the current 50 percent. They made a business case for the redesigned joint care program that brought together the financial gains from the proposed changes (lower costs as a result of fewer inpatient days, etc.) and the investments needed to realize the necessary medical improvements. This way, hospital management realized they could reduce costs by about €700 per patient, achieving a total net increase in profits of about €600,000 (based on estimates of the number of patients treated).[2]

During the annual negotiation with the largest insurance company, which has a market share of roughly 70 percent in this southern region, the CEO of the Atrium Medical Center took a considerable risk. He put the business case right out on the table and revealed not just the gains of the redesigned trajectory but also the total cost for Atrium to provide the treatment. The insurance company appreciated his openness and proposed an agreement making the Atrium Medical Center the "preferred partner" for knee and hip replacements in the region. The insurer would send all its clients a letter indicating that the Atrium Medical Center was the place to go for knee or hip replacement. The insurer supported and participated in the festive opening of the center for elective treatment that the Atrium Medical Center organized some months after the negotiations. The insurer and the hospital decided on a price that gave the Atrium Medical Center a reasonable profit for offering joint care at a substantially lower price than neighboring hospitals.

The director was satisfied with this "golden deal." The risk he had taken by putting all his cards on the table seemed to have paid off. But the quality manager, who was supposed to coordinate the innovation process, still had a major concern. The business case was still based on *proposed* changes, not on achieved results. Though it may have been easy to sell this product at such a low price, she knew that it would not be easy to transform the improved care process from a plan into a reality. She wondered whether the "done deal" would help to achieve the necessary changes, or whether the orthopedic department would be facing a financial deficit the next year.

Dynamic Relationships Between Market Mechanisms and Delivery of Health Care

Concerns about the relationship between health care delivery and market mechanisms have a long history. Even Adam Smith argued, in *The Wealth of Nations*, that the invisible hand would be an imperfect mechanism when used to regulate health care.[3] The trust that patients should invest in their doctors and the importance of medical professionals' receiving solid education would sit uneasily with a doctor's need for income unless such wages were protected through restricted admission to the medical profession (Smith 1776, chapter X).[4]

More than 200 years later, exploring and reconfiguring those very limitations of free market mechanisms in health care has become the daily business of health economists. The founding father of health economics, Kenneth Arrow, supposed that "when the market fails to achieve an optimal state, society will, to some extent at least, recognize the gap and nonmarket social institutions will arise attempting to bridge it" (1963, p. 947).[5] Ever since, health economists have largely focused on the study and development of those "social institutions" and on how health economics can contribute to the construction of these "optimal states." As a result, health economists have focused much of their practical and theoretical efforts on constructing a health care market that does not depend on an "invisible hand" ascertaining public values once health care markets are "deregulated," but that is built upon the notion developed by health economists of "regulated" or "managed competition" (Enthoven 1988; Enthoven and van de Ven 2007).

Policy makers, policy scientists, and health economists have been increasingly collaborating in designing market-based health policy programs and putting them into practice. Whereas in the late 1980s Malcolm Ashmore, Michael Mulkay, and Trevor Pinch still saw health economists as marginalized players and underdogs relative to clinicians and policy makers (1989), today such economists are major policy actors, populating influential regulatory agencies throughout Western policy systems (van Egmond and Zuiderent-Jerak 2010). Health economics is therefore heavily involved in the construction of markets for public values, and the practices through which these goals are pursued have gradually become topics of analytical and normative interest for researchers from other fields (Ashmore, Mulkay, and Pinch 1989; Sjögren and Helgesson 2007; Grit and Dolfsma 2002).

Unfortunately, the structure of the present debate on marketization in health care threatens to restrict the space for empirical study. There are clear and often ideological divisions between protagonists of health care markets who claim that providing "incentives" for competition automatically ensures efficiency in health care and critics who claim that the managerialization of health care is ruining the actual work professionals carry out. The claim that markets can still be kept away from health care (Godlee 2006) or the claim that health care "is not a market" (Palm 2005) leaves unaddressed crucial questions about the specific consequences of market mechanisms for the improvement of health care. These questions include how market mechanisms in health care are made to work, which "others" are constituted in the newly created market "orders" (Berg and Timmermans 2000), and what potential alternative configurations of market mechanisms can be envisioned. Such questions may be too important for the development and study of market mechanisms to be left entirely to health economists and policy makers.

How Economics Performs Markets and May Be Getting Company

In recent years, the social study of markets has undergone challenging theoretical developments through the work of Michel Callon and colleagues (Callon 1998a–c, 1999; Callon and Muniesa 2005; Callon, Méadel, and Rabeharisoa 2002; Barry and Slater 2002b; Callon, Millo, and Muniesa 2007). Callon and his co-authors addressed "the performativity of economics" (MacKenzie and Millo 2003; MacKenzie, Muniesa, and Siu 2007). After early work in actor-network theory (ANT) about how scientific facts are produced and enacted through *hybrid collectifs* (Callon and Law 1995) in which scientists play a crucial role (Latour and Woolgar 1979; Latour 1987; Callon 1986), Callon turned his attention to economics. Consistent with ANT studies of the natural sciences, he argued that economics not only discovers independently existing market laws but is actively involved in bringing those laws into being. This empirical turn allows for a study of how markets are performed through the activities of economists and has opened up the enactment of markets for empirical scrutiny, creating "an abundance of ways of *seeing* economic markets" (Barry and Slater 2002b, p. 291).

According to Callon (1998b, p. 51), this empirical turn not only has theoretical and analytical implications; it is also highly consequential for the roles social scientists may play in the *reconfiguration* of emerging markets:

The market is no longer that cold, implacable and impersonal monster which imposes its laws and procedures while extending them ever further. It is a many-sided, diversified, evolving device which the social sciences as well as the actors themselves contribute to reconfigure.

In the light of the often-polarized debate on the marketization of health care, Callon's work can be taken as an important reminder that "it would be a mistake to be simply opposed to markets or to marketization" (Callon in Barry and Slater 2002a, p. 186). This warning against sociological anti-market sentimentality allows one to raise the question of how markets are reconfigured by various actors. This creates important space for researchers in social studies of markets to explore particular forms of markets—thereby challenging the monopoly on this topic from health policy makers and economists.

The focus on the performativity of economics also opens up "markets as political issues" which can either be studied critically or, as Callon proposes, reconfigured actively through "experimenting with new configurations" (ibid., p. 288). *How* to do such reconfiguration is, unfortunately, empirically and conceptually under-explored, which makes it quite relevant to put Callon's proposals to the market test.

In this chapter I will explore how Callon's work relates to social-science research on and intervention in the experimental development of health care markets in the Netherlands. Therefore, I now turn to the project in which I was actively involved as one of the "innovative actors [who] are experimenting with new configurations" (Callon in Barry and Slater 2002b, p. 288) of health care markets.

Improvement and Marketization of Health Care: The Case of Better Faster

In November 2003 the Dutch Ministry of Health, Welfare and Sport, together with the Dutch Hospital Association, launched a large initiative called Better Faster. The initiative explicitly aimed to improve the quality, the safety, and the efficiency of the hospital care sector. It also was widely perceived as a demonstration of the Ministry's willingness to invest in quality at a time of dramatic change in health policy associated with the introduction of regulated competition for Dutch health care. In the following two years, the Ministry began switching its payment structure to a system based on diagnosis-related groups, which (as was mentioned above) was designed to set up price competition for a percentage of DRGs. The Ministry also introduced the new health insurance law that was supposed to help insurance companies become ever-more-powerful players in negotiating the price and the quality of health care. The initiative largely resonated with the aims of the broader changes in the policy of regulated competition. The main assumption of the initiative was that health care delivery can "often be done faster or better"—

Faster, because care must be available when it is needed. Better, because it needs to be as safe, efficient and patient-friendly as possible. That is why we need to be more open about how we use both human and financial resources. We need to make it easier to compare the performance of care providers. So they need to work on the basis of clear norms and protocols. And good practice needs to be applied faster. After all, care providers have a lot to learn from each other. (Ministry of Health Welfare and Sport 2005)

The initiative covered a range of activities that, it was said, would "prepare the hospital sector for the new care system" (ibid.).

The Better Faster initiative consisted of three "pillars." The first was a set of activities aimed at increasing awareness of good practices, partly through an online "best practice" database and partly through "ambassadors" from large business firms who presented their views on such matters as safety, logistics, and accountability in health care. As part of the work in this pillar, Rein Willems, then CEO of Shell Royal Dutch Oil, asserted that his company's slogan "You work safely or you don't work here at all" (Shell Nederland 2004) was equally applicable to the health care sector, which needed to have a safety-management system up and running in a few years. Peter Bakker, the CEO of TPG, a large logistics firm that includes the recently privatized Dutch postal service, stated that "2.5 billion euros" could be saved in the hospital sector through logistic improvements (TPG 2004).

In January of 2004 the Dutch Healthcare Inspectorate introduced the second pillar: a set of performance indicators for hospital care, which was to be extended and improved upon in the coming years.[6] The third pillar was a quality, innovation, and efficiency collaborative initiated in October 2004. It was set up in three tiers of eight hospitals, with each hospital included for two years at a stretch and each group starting one year after the previous one. Hospitals had to apply for inclusion in the program and, once selected, would not have to pay for participation in the collaborative. Interestingly, this ministerial choice was challenged by health care consultancies, which claimed that investing in quality by assigning advisors to hospitals and allowing them to participate in the collaborative without having to pay for it was a form of market contamination. The Ministry compromised by hiring some of these consultants as advisors who would be assigned to hospitals.

The Better Faster initiative consisted of a package of projects to be carried out by each participating hospital. The projects included preventing post-operative wound infections, preventing bed sores, making the operating room more efficient, reducing medication errors, installing blame-free reporting, providing instant access to outpatient clinics, redesigning processes for oncology care and elective surgery, and improving the leadership of hospital management. In this third pillar, national working conferences were held for the participating hospital teams on each improvement theme, and each hospital received substantial support through these conferences and by being assigned an advisor who spent several days a week working on the various projects and advising unit management and the board of directors.

The three pillars of the Better Faster program were supposed to reinforce one another and to encourage participating actors to compete for efficiency and high quality:

The aim is to help parties in the field improve their performance, starting with hospital and primary health care, where there is plenty of room for improvement. The programme does not only target care providers, since it is important for as many parties as possible to benefit from the activities being implemented under its aegis. It will help insurers, for instance, to see who is and who isn't adopting proven good practice. (Ministry of Health Welfare and Sport 2005)

Better Faster was a highly layered set-up, using benchmarking to classify differences between hospitals, performance indicators to monitor practices, and the collaborative improvement program to substantially enhance patient safety and patient logistics.

Contrary to the idea that regulated competition is a system that can be "implemented," the Better Faster initiative can be seen as *performing health care as a market of a particular kind*: a market in which actors would not simply compete over the *price* of the "care products" or the *service levels*, but where negotiations between hospitals and insurance companies about the price paid for health care products would include a similar focus on increasing medical quality and patient-centeredness. The initiative could be analyzed as a set of experimental devices to materialize the notion that competition in health care should aim to "increase value"—an aim that would probably not be achieved simply by starting a price war (Porter and Olmsted Teisberg 2004). For example, speakers at conferences on medication safety emphasized that reducing the number of administered blood transfusions is both a safety issue for patients and a major cost-saving instrument. Some of my colleagues from the Institute of Health Policy and Management produced a study (Manna et al. 2006) that reconfigured pressure ulcers from a *quality* issue to a *major cost issue*, as ulcer treatment would require much longer hospitalization that would no longer produce revenue for hospitals in the new payment structure. Whereas previously they had received a fee per inpatient day, they were now being paid a fixed fee for a care trajectory, which explains why extra costs incurred by longer hospitalization did not produce more revenue. "Inpatient days" was no longer a category in the accounts receivable budgeting system, but was now a *cost* that hospitals would have to deduct from their income. Through such initiatives, the actors in the collaborative tried to connect cost-saving possibilities to organizational ways of making care patient-centered. Preventing pressure ulcers was not merely based on the normative appeal to treat patients in the most suitable way; it was a direct part of the business model of the hospital.

The Institute of Health, Policy and Management at Erasmus University Rotterdam was heavily involved in the second and third pillars of the Better Faster initiative. Researchers from that institute were responsible for developing a set of indicators, following a highly experimental and pragmatic strategy in a debate on performance indicators that had long been dominated by scientistic issues of validation and accuracy.[7] The institute was also one of the three consortium partners running the third pillar. (The other two partners were the Dutch Institute for Healthcare Improvement and the Netherlands Association of Medical Specialists.) Because of my experience with pathwaying projects in the university hospital discussed in the preceding chapters, I ended up as the national project leader of the process-redesign project and as a hospital advisor for the Atrium Medical Center.[8]

Pathwaying and the Cost of Poor Quality

The project to redesign care processes prominently articulated the notion that creating high-quality patient-centered care was not just a quality-improvement strategy but also could be used as a "business strategy." The notion of "situated standardization" as a sociological contribution to health care improvement was also put at center stage in this national project, and the need for standards situated in sociologically articulated issues soon also proved valuable. Teams collaborating on the improvement project were required to produce overviews of appointments, diagnostic activities, treatments, and follow-up procedures. These overviews had to be based on trajectories patients actually followed, not ideal typical pathways. For each item, a date had to be recorded to enable insight into the duration of the trajectories. As I described in the introduction to this book, one of the multidisciplinary groups improving care for patients with colon and rectum carcinoma found that patients were receiving colonoscopies more often than was medically necessary. Even when a gastroenterologist had performed a colonoscopy and had diagnosed colon cancer, a surgeon would subsequently perform the same colonoscopy with a static scope rather than the flexible one used in initial diagnostics. The gastroenterologist had not been aware of the duplicated procedure before the overview.

In discussing this finding in the project group, Dr. Jan Roijers, the surgical oncologist group member, pointed out that Dr. Maarten Pols and his colleagues in the gastroenterology department did not register the distance between the anus and the tumor with sufficient accuracy, when this was crucial for deciding on treatment. If a tumor was situated in the last 12–15 cm of the large intestine, it was defined as a case of rectum carcinoma to be treated with a combination of radiation therapy and resection. When situated elsewhere it was defined as colon carcinoma, which would not require radiation therapy but swift resection instead. Dr. Pols and colleagues were unaware of the importance of this precise tumor location, and this had led to unpleasant surprises for surgeons who only found out *during an operation* that they should have given radiation therapy before surgery. Since mortality for treatment of rectum carcinoma without radiation therapy is higher, they were in fact reducing the patient's chances of survival. Once the surgeons learned that data produced by gastroenterologists were "unreliable," they began to perform their own colonoscopies with patients diagnosed with colon cancer, to define the exact position of the tumor. The meeting of the improvement team led to a change in the gastroenterologists' practice, to ensure that they would register a tumor's location precisely. Consequently, patients did not have to undergo the unpleasant colonoscopy procedure twice, which also lowered the risk of infection from the procedure. This enhanced effectiveness, since treating the cancer did not have to be postponed until after the second colonoscopy; it also improved efficiency, since it no longer wasted costly diagnostic tests and physicians' valuable time.

Quality improvement through inter-professional collaboration is, in itself, nothing new; stories about the sometimes striking simplicity of quality improvement abound. It is the aim of the Quality Improvement Collaboratives run by the US Institute for Healthcare Improvement, and of other quality forums. Within Better Faster, however, providing safe and rapid treatment was not merely seen as a gain for patients or a matter of professional responsibility by practitioners; it was also presented as a viable business strategy within an emerging market for hospital care. Because this is a far from common way of positioning quality initiatives, it is worth exploring *how* health care improvement was enacted as business strategy for competing hospitals. And according to Callon, social scientists can learn something from health economists in this regard:

The weakness of sociology and anthropology when they come to analyse economic activities is precisely their reluctance to do the same jobs as economics. Economists are able to tell how it is possible to calculate profits and so on, but sociologists do not provide these kinds of tools ... [we should] devise our own tools, like the economists, but tools that will endow economics agents with the capacity to experiment with different forms of markets organization (Callon in Barry and Slater 2002b, pp. 300-301).

Because of the importance of metrication practices for both the hemophilia care center and the hematology/oncology ward, particularly when looking at differences in treatment patterns and experimenting with the introduction of temperature loggers or measuring how late surgery was running, I recognized right away that we needed tools for calculating quality improvement. Within the project team for re-designing care processes,[9] we focused on calculations that would produce overviews of patient trajectories and of the activities carried out in various phases. We set two generic goals for improvement projects: a decrease of 40–90 percent in throughput time for all care trajectories and a decrease of 30 percent in length of stay for all care processes that include hospitalization. We believed that these goals would increase the chance of identifying both inefficiencies that were equally harmful to patients and to hospitals. In addition, we were not too concerned whether those goals would be met; we thought of them mainly as devices to frame reflexivity (van Loon and Zuiderent-Jerak 2012) and to permit hospitals to think radically and creatively about possibilities for improving their patient trajectories. We were quite sure that reducing throughput time and length of stay would be important, since these measures so often pointed to other matters of poor coordination leading to unnecessary suffering. Yet the exact goals were set rather haphazardly. I had been receiving emails on the aims of the process-redesign project, because the Ministry wanted the program to go live with clear targets for all projects. Because I could not quite see how we should decide what a suitable target would be, I had tried to ignore these messages as long as I could. As the deadline for delivering the project's aims approached, the program manager called me just as I was boarding a commuter train. Then and there, I told him what our targets would be, based on some initial thoughts we had had on the project team, and pretty much decided them on the spot. To my surprise, these targets were never challenged by the program manager, the Ministry, or the participating hospitals—not even the rather wide range of the first target.

As participating hospitals selected many different diseases for their patient trajectories, the improvement teams were encouraged to formulate

specific goals on quality, efficiency, and patient-centeredness, in addition
to the generic goals. To monitor whether project aims were achieved *and* as
an intervention in the improvement projects, measuring throughput times
became crucial. We therefore introduced a measurement tool that would
register the steps in patient trajectories and tabulate average durations for
each step.[10] (See figure 4.2.)

This measurement tool performed care trajectories in particular ways.
First, by separating the trajectory into various phases, such as "admission
time to outpatient clinic," "diagnostic trajectory," and "length of stay," it
articulated specific problems in the organization of care. Second, by displaying the median and the average of each indicator, it indicated whether the
process was highly variable or fairly similar for particular groups of patients.
Third, adding indicators such as "number of visits prior to treatment" articulated how diagnostic procedures could be combined in a single visit (called
"one-stop shopping diagnostics" in the jargon of health care improvement),
or, as in the case of the double colonoscopies, how they could be eliminated.

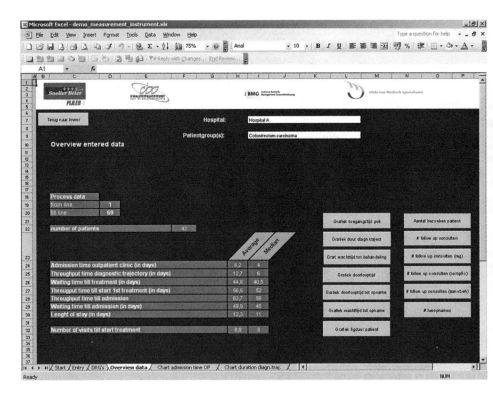

Figure 4.2
Measurement instrument for process redesign

To further support the notion that project gains could be realized by reducing the number of steps, all teams were asked to do what I had done at the hematology/oncology outpatient clinic: produce "flow charts" of the care processes on which they were working. Combining these charts with the calculated waiting time for each individual step or phase in the process connected quality of care, throughput time, and number of activities. At the same time, the flow charts remained sketchy, glossing over many details of *exactly what* should happen in each individual step in the care process. To emphasize that flow charts should articulate issues and generate quality improvement, rather than be representations of medical work that care professionals should adhere to, I asked teams to draw intentionally sketchy flow charts. Utilizing this approach, I tried to accommodate the notion of situated standardization developed in previous projects. This pragmatic and sociologically inspired way of doing standardization caused some frustration among quality managers who had been formally trained in the development and introduction of integrated care pathways and who had learned to map and describe each step in the care process, redesign it, and implement it—exactly the kind of separation of innovation and implementation that I fervently tried to avoid. At the same time, it caused enthusiasm among care professionals who had become increasingly frustrated by the rigidity and level of detail of integrated care pathways and who liked the focus of standardizing only the aspects that they actually experienced as problematic and the aspects for which they felt it would contribute to a solution.

The charts often focused on issues that had also come up in previous projects. The preparation of intake visits turned out to be a problem in many hospitals, leading to frustrating experiences for care professionals and patients alike. Extra visits were a burden on outpatient clinics but also on patients, who needed to pay more hospital visits than necessary, and wait longer than needed before treatment could start. In processes like the one described for gall bladder removal (see figure 4.3) or other small surgical procedures, the pre-operative consult with the anesthetist often turned out to cause long delays. After the consult with the surgeon, patients were referred to the anesthetist for their pre-operative checkup. Waiting for the appointment could easily take a few weeks, after which the anesthetist would assess the risk of complications. Only then could an appointment for the surgery be made, which could easily take yet another few weeks. All this made the whole process for small elective surgical procedures take far too long. Several participating hospitals focused on these kinds of processes. At the Atrium Medical Center, the initial measurement of throughput times for patient trajectories shocked all those who were involved. The total time

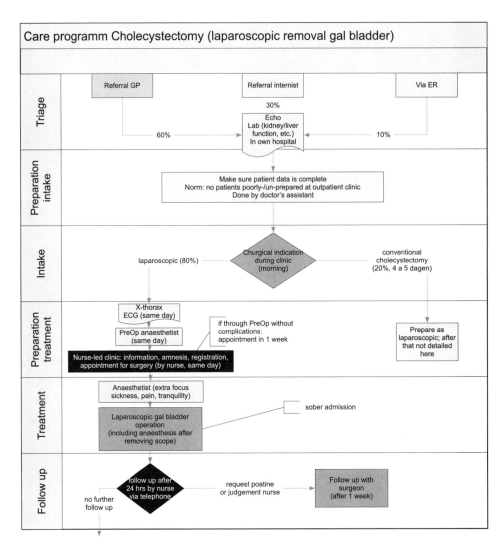

Figure 4.3
Flow chart for laparoscopic gall bladder removal.

from referral by a general practitioner to discharge after follow-up was, on average, 94½ days—more than three months—for very minor procedures. The time patients had to wait from referral till treatment was, on average, 68 days. About half that time was spent waiting after referral by the general practitioner and 33 days by extra visits for diagnostic consults and for the anesthetist's pre-operative checkup. These months of waiting did not necessarily lead to an aggravation of patients' health status, but they did result in unnecessary discomfort, inability to perform societal responsibilities, and (potentially) use of sick leave.

Throughput time was increased further because the operating surgeon saw all patients in follow-up visits. As was described in the introduction to this book, I asked Dr. Hans Brakema (the surgeon heading the improvement team) whether follow-up visits really were necessary for small surgical procedures. He got quite upset and replied "I truly think it is unethical if I plunged a knife into someone's body and never shook their hand afterwards!" To some extent I agreed with him, but I did wonder if it was more unethical to have patients wait longer before getting access to a surgeon because surgery hours were filled up with follow-up visits. Fortunately, each of the project teams had an external advisor and an advisor from the hospital's quality-management department. The quality manager of this hospital, Ingrid Joosen, made a suggestion that I did not understand at the time: "Why don't we find out from our hospital information system how often a surgeon who carries out the operation actually does the follow-up?" This turned out to be a not-so-innocent guess. She knew that the partnership of surgeons had developed an unspoken division of labor over the years for the simple reason that some surgeons were highly efficient in the operating theater, whereas others were better at doing surgery hours than their colleagues. Out of necessity, and despite their sincere normative attachments to good care, these specialists had come to accept that some colleagues would spend more time in the outpatient clinic and others would spend more time in the operating room. This meant that even though patients had follow-up visits with the surgeon who had seen them before their operation, it did not necessarily mean that this would be the same person who had "plunged the knife" into their bodies. Since these figures were not a standard part of the measurement tool, extra metrication was required. But once that metrication was done, we found out that there was a match between the operating surgeon and the one doing the follow-up in no more than 5 percent of all surgical procedures.

We discussed this finding in the working group. Ingrid Joosen and I agreed with the normative claim about surgeons seeing the patients they had operated on, but we felt that this applied particularly to oncological patients, for whom it mattered enormously what a surgeon had seen during the operation. Such patients tend to be full of questions about the level of metastasis, how far the tumor had stuck to or grown into surrounding organs, and how clean the cut was (a good indicator of the chances that a tumor was fully removed). Besides that, there may be patients who do not share the ethical concerns of this surgeon. They may think it fine not having to come in for follow-up if there are no complications, as they wouldn't have to take time off from work or arrange backup care for their children. So we proposed to free up the space in the surgery hours and effectuate this laudable principle in severe surgical cases, but not in others. We drew up a checklist of questions about possible complications that nurses would ask in a telephone call the day after the operation. If the nurses established that there was no immediate clinical reason for having a face-to-face follow-up, they would always finish by asking whether the patient had any other questions, doubts, or uncertainties and whether he or she would still like to see a doctor. We estimated that about 20 percent of patients requiring follow-up because of complications or because they still wanted to see a doctor, which freed up 80 percent of the visits now dedicated to follow-up. Nurses were trained in working with the checklist and took care of this in their clinic. Since general practitioners were informed about the new working method and explained it to patients in advance, and since the nurses calling postoperative patients had already seen them on the day of their operation and had reminded them that they would call the next day, most patients did indeed feel fine with not coming back to the hospital for follow-up, and our estimate of 20 percent was quite accurate. Furthermore, Ingrid Joosen worked with the IT department to set up a monthly query for Dr. Brakema to keep track of the matches between operating surgeons and surgeons performing follow-up.

Not only was the situated standardization approach more workable than the more rigorous approach of developing integrated care pathways, some interventions could work *only* because they were not based on the ICP niche standardization approach. A direct-access pre-operative anesthetist surgery hour cannot be established for a select patient group, as it is simply not possible to have an anesthetist on standby for this separate group. The alternative of reserving slots for such patients would be detrimental to the overall productivity of anesthetists, as these slots might not get filled. But changing the working method in the anesthesiology department so that *all elective patients* had direct access began to pay off. Other interventions, such as the nurse-led clinic to prepare patients better and free up time in doctors' surgery hours, were started for some groups of patients, but nurses and surgeons soon began wondering why more patient groups weren't included, and they scaled up such interventions rapidly.

In the case of the Atrium Medical Center, these improvements resulted in substantial changes to the throughput time of elective surgical procedures. The total trajectory used to be more than three months, but now it was down to seven days in all for the large majority of patients: five days of access time from the time of referral by the general practitioner; one day for the intake with the surgeon, the visit in the nurse-led clinic, a visit to the anesthetist, and surgery in the afternoon, and—on the seventh day, after the operation—the nurse's follow-up phone call. This was a 93 percent reduction in throughput time, which meant we had managed to exceed the process-redesign project's general target of a reduction ranging from 40 percent to 90 percent. Moreover, it implied a deduction from an average 4.8 outpatient clinic visits per patient to 1.2 visits for the large majority of patients: one visit for the day of surgery, and 0.2 visits for the 20 percent of patients that still needed or wanted a face-to-face follow-up consult. This meant an overall 75 percent reduction in outpatient clinic visits. The number of inpatient days, formerly 3.2, was now less than one—a reduction of 69 percent.

Exceeding the project's aims in these improvement initiatives was a very welcome surprise, in view of my initial insecurity about these targets. I was not just worried whether they would make sense to care professionals or be challenged as absurd and unfeasible. When asked to set the project targets, I had feared that meeting the aims might become more important than safeguarding intelligent and skillfully developed care practices already in existence. I was concerned that embracing "the novel" too enthusiastically might harm existing good care that would become functionally invisible in these ambitious improvement projects. (See chapters 1 and 3.) Interestingly, and in line with my findings in previous projects, I found that scholarly attachments to invisible work may develop too easily into the sentimental idea that *all* social action is skillful and reflexive. Many of the practices within these improvement teams were either based on sympathetic but *problematic* reflections (as in the case of surgical follow-up for small elective procedures) or based on a perhaps organized *lack* of interprofessional reflection.

Furthermore, I felt that skillful invisible work was partly safeguarded by the approach of situated standardization that left untouched many parts of practice that were not seen as problematic. The combination of sketchy flow charts and improvised measurement tools began to enact the delivery of health care as part of a coordinated process rather than as activities split into separate episodes and disciplines, and it allowed for process standardization in a way roomy enough for complexity and variation in the case of individual patients and for instances in which standardization would not be a solution to an empirically specified problem. For example, we did not address what surgeons discussed during their surgery hours or what activities nurses carried out when caring for patients. This approach was crucial to involving professionals in the improvement agenda. Some enthusiastic doctors adopted and modified the metrication tools, using the relatively simple features of Microsoft Excel to calculate the inter-doctor variability for certain aspects of care. In a presentation based on such modifications, a vascular surgeon at a national working conference told some 200 colleagues from 16 hospitals about the different steps patients with the same disease had to go through in his hospital. He stated that he and his fellow surgeons had found no medically valid explanation for the differences in their practices, and that this had led them to do something they hadn't done for quite a while: discuss how to deliver the best care most efficiently.

The other members of the care-process-redesign team and I were, of course, pleased with these instances of quality improvement. To enact these developments as part of the introduction of health care markets, however, we still had to show how *financially* interesting the improvements were. Thus, contributing to the configuration of a health care market in which quality improvement, rather than price and high "service levels," was an important business strategy for the Better Faster hospitals. Cooperation with both health economists and financial analysts in hospitals was extremely fruitful for developing "business cases" for redesigned care trajectories (Leatherman et al. 2003). Rather than assuming that "economists, by profession, tend to think in terms of a tug of war between the private sector and public sector" (Callon in Barry and Slater 2002b, p. 299), I learned that the cliché that economists are against regulation is even less applicable to *health* economists than to other economists. As was explained above, health care has always had a *status aparte* in discussions about the "free" market. But even when discussing economics at large, I would suggest that the very idea that economists monopolize discussions of potential market forms is a consequence of the distance economic sociologists and anthropologists *and* Callon have created between themselves and economics. Situated-intervention involvements with other scientific practices have shown that other disciplines often turn out to be "far from unified and in fact highly contested internally[,] the strongest critique … com[ing] from within the discipline" (Kember 2003, p. 176). Those of us who were involved with the project team working to re-design care processes preferred the approach of "engaging strategically with the differences within [economics]" (Kember 2002, p. 638) rather than "rehearsing endless critiques of conventional economics and often in a vain attempt, a delusion, that [we] might convince economists" (Callon in Barry and Slater 2002b, p. 301). This stance meant that our team could receive substantial help from some of the participating hospitals and from health economists at the Institute of Health Policy and Management. Input from the financial departments of individual hospitals proved useful in articulating the financial gains from redesigned care trajectories. I soon found out that financial employees were busily calculating cost per step in care processes while working far from the actual process of care delivery—generally in a hospital's basement. Until recently, hospitals had no need to know the costs of their various activities. The financial structure of the hospital used to focus mainly on interventions and activities that generated income, and on the cost, in a more general sense, of personnel, equipment, and so forth. As part of the introduction of the new funding system in which insurance companies paid a fixed fee for an entire care trajectory, it became all the more important for hospital management and doctors to know the costs of *all the work* that was carried out in these care processes: otherwise they could be selling care processes at a loss. This need to know the costs of care processes resulted in members of the financial staff working overtime to produce financial information for items that had never had a price before. These monetary calculations enabled improvement teams to calculate the financial benefits of a well-organized care trajectory. Teams could combine the costs of the steps presented in the overview tool and develop a business case that individually priced existing and desired processes, thus rendering "the cost of poor quality" visible. (See figure 4.4.)

Accordingly, for one hospital the new trajectory for patients with colon or rectum carcinoma resulted in a difference of approximately €950 per patient on a total cost of less than €5,500. This came partly from savings achieved by stopping duplicate colonoscopies, but it was mainly generated by the introduction of a new protocol that was under development in international studies on colorectal cancer treatment: the enhanced recovery after surgery (ERAS) protocol. This protocol, which had been tested for some years (Willmore and Kehlet 2001), was later tested more widely (Fearong et al. 2005). It was mainly a combination of careful pain management, anesthesia practices focused on preventing postoperative nausea, and dietary practices that differed from those commonly practiced. In common practice, a patient whose bowels have been operated on needs a long rest, should be cautious about eating, and generally has too much pain to start eating in the first place. The downside of this is that the patient's condition deteriorates rapidly because he spends several days in bed with little food. If pain is managed carefully, if nausea is prevented by medication, and if a regular diet is resumed as soon as is possible, the patient has to recover only from the surgery and not from physical deterioration caused by days of inaction and fasting.

fin.code	activity	profile baseline				desired process	
		frequency	price/unit	costs		frequency	costs
190011	Intake visit internist/GE	1,00	€ 33,15	€ 33,15		1,00	€ 33,15
411000	Return visit internist/GE	2,21	€ 26,52	€ 58,61		0,50	€ 13,26
190011	Intake visit surgeon	1,00	€ 30,19	€ 30,19		1,00	€ 30,19
411000	Return visit surgeon	0,69	€ 24,15	€ 16,66		0,10	€ 2,42
190011	Intake visit cardiology	0,17	€ 27,21	€ 4,63		0,17	€ 4,63
411000	Return visit cardiology	0,17	€ 21,77	€ 3,70		0,17	€ 3,70
	Pre-Op	1,07					
190035	Day treatment	1,02	€ 151,92	€ 154,96		1,00	€ 151,92
34686	Colonoscopy	0,89	€ 253,01	€ 225,18		1,00	€ 253,01
34690	Sigmoidscopy	0,22	€ 204,90	€ 45,08		0,05	€ 10,25
39876	Rectoscopy	0,46	€ 125,60	€ 57,78		0,00	
50501	Biopt (PA)	1,06	€ 42,94	€ 45,52		1,06	€ 45,52
87511	X-colon	0,30	€ 148,00	€ 44,40		0,15	€ 22,20
85002	X-thorax	1,02	€ 43,44	€ 44,31		1,00	€ 43,44
87090	MRI Abdomen	0,44	€ 278,84	€ 122,69		0,66	€ 184,03
87070	Echo stomach organs	0,80	€ 92,30	€ 73,84		0,66	€ 60,92
39494	Echo heart	0,09	€ 53,00	€ 4,77		0,09	€ 4,77
87042	CT abdomen	0,06	€ 235,12	€ 14,11		0,00	
07-_-_	Lab			€ 102,38			€ 102,38
34738	Colon resection	0,60	€ 1.542,00	€ 925,20		0,60	€ 925,20
35024	Anterior resection	0,35	€ 2.057,00	€ 719,95		0,35	€ 719,95
34732	Total colectomy	0,05	€ 2.814,00	€ 140,70		0,05	€ 140,70
	Inpatient						
190204	Inpatient days	12,30	€ 206,04	€ 2.534,29		7,00	€ 1.442,28
			Total: hard euro's	**€ 5.402,08**		Total: soft euro's	**€ 4.193,91**

Figure 4.4
Business case for colon/rectum carcinoma.

The surgeons had followed the international literature on the ERAS protocol but until now had felt reluctant to try the new way of working in their own hospital. They were still following the discussion of potential risks for higher readmission rates and late complications, but were also worried about the nurses' reactions to substantial changes in the intensive care unit. But now, in the project, they were willing to try the ERAS protocol, as it seemed promising for reducing the length of stay. Patients could have shorter hospitalizations with lower infection risks, which would release pressure on inpatient wards and nursing staff. Nurses in the ICU were indeed highly suspicious of this change, and they were worried that the process would be far too demanding for patients. They were all the more surprised when some patients began asking if they could get out of bed even while they were still in the ICU recovering from the surgery.

For small elective surgical procedures, the 75 percent reduction in visits to the outpatient clinic, the reduction in inpatient days, and the surgeons' time saved added up to a cost reduction of €379 per patient. The investment needed to let nurses make the follow-up phone call and have doctors' assistants chase patient data to prevent poorly prepared intake visits was just over €5 per patient. The differences were not due entirely to the difference in tariffs between doctors and nurses or doctors' assistants. One important factor probably is that cost assessments were based on formal representations of work, which tend to be more detailed and inclusive for doctors than for other professionals whose work is largely invisible (Suchman 1995; Star 1991a). However, in this case the invisibility of nursing work had an advantage in that it allowed for a stronger connection between the organization of care and costs that made quality improvement very attractive for the management in this hospital.

The development of these calculative devices proved highly consequential. The approach was adopted widely by many sites, including the Atrium Medical Center. Soon after the first results came in, an Atrium board member presented the expected outcomes of the redesign projects to his management team in both qualitative and financial terms. His presentation had the telling title Return to the Essence: Top Quality Care with Maximum Profit. This session led hospital management to embrace the redesign of care processes as their main strategy for the coming two years, with the aim of redesigning care for at least 50 percent of patients in that period. The hospital's director gave a similar presentation at a national working conference of the project to redesign care processes.

At the Atrium Medical Center, the consequences of treating quality improvement and financial matters together also manifested in an interesting discussion about assigning new members of the nursing staff to elective surgery. I witnessed it take place between the hospital's director and a manager of one of its three branches. Having presented the business case for a cluster of smaller surgical procedures, such as laparoscopic removal of gall bladders and inguinal hernias, the hospital's director said that the location manager could simply submit a proposal for extra nursing staff, since he had worked out a perfect business case to cover the investment. "Just hand it in to me and I'll pass it through the board meeting next week without any problems," said the director. "But I don't need to," the location manager replied. "I'm showing that I can cover the investment in extra nursing time with the gains we get from improving the process. And I still have nursing hours left over!"

Both to the actors involved and to me as an advisor witnessing the interaction, it was unusual to hear a manager refuse such an offer, and it was easy to imagine how different the conversation would have been without these calculative devices. That financial costs and quality gains can be subject to unexpected relationships once they are brought together in a calculative space seems to confirm Callon's proposal. By articulating the delivery of care as a process, it became possible to recombine elements in such a way that work that was previously seen as a cost was now being seen as an investment. The introduction of a nurse-led clinic for patients undergoing elective surgical interventions would, when assessed in isolation, be treated as a cost—as one step in the care-delivery process. Now, treating the various steps together enabled improvement agents to treat it as an investment in one phase of the process that produced savings in later phases.

With some reservations, I could say that we were successful in helping to set up a health care market in which actors competed on "value" rather than on price and service delivery. Experimentally creating collective calculative devices interwove quality improvements and financial gains, and health professionals were potentially disabused of their historically justified fears of budget cuts. Drawing together doctors, flow charts, health economists, financial analysts, follow-up ratios, DRG pricing systems, sociological intervention scholars, Excel spreadsheets, colonoscopies, and processual insights in this redesign initiative resulted in a practice that performed an alternative market that had nothing to do with health care's *adhering* to abstract market mechanisms but instead had to do with actively *reconfiguring a specific kind of market in this health care setting.*

"If we accept that there is nothing which could happen without being framed," Barry and Slater (2002b) quote Callon as having said, "the role of the sociology and anthropology of economies is precisely to design tools and to provide actors with such tools." At some point in this project, however, I began to realize that such an exclusive focus on designing and providing such tools, as one of the main "performative activities of the social sciences" (ibid.), could prove to be a limited and tricky strategy. Callon ascribes a crucial role to the construction of calculative devices, but in this case there seemed to be a more dynamic relation between market activity and the availability and functioning of market instruments.

Fragile Devices, Robust Markets

According to Callon, the most important asset of actor-network theory is that it "is based on no stable theory of the actor; rather it assumes the *radical indeterminacy* of the actor" (1999, p. 181). The main advantage of this redistribution of agency is that it opens up the social sciences to non-humans, so that it becomes possible to show the importance of technologies for performing markets in specific ways. In this case, spaces of calculation were created through interaction with Excel spreadsheets, flow charts, project meetings, hospital information systems, national quality-improvement collaboratives, and hospital boardrooms. Market practices in health care were performed in ways that added value in accordance with the vision for hospitals as organizations striving for a balance of public values. Following the strategy of "drawing things together" (Latour 1990), associating and disassociating the relevant actors seemed to produce suitable calculative devices for reconfiguring marketized health care as value-driven.

It was both interesting and puzzling to experience how *easy* it was, relatively speaking, to reconfigure a health care market based on cost saving and service level into a value-driven one. It certainly did not happen without effort, but was it really feasible to perform this shift simply by creating calculative devices? Making these devices available would not seem sufficient to endow the respective calculative spaces with impressive agency, since relations between "high quality" and "competitive advantage" were often loose, ambiguous, and susceptible to serious challenge from strong actors. For example, the new Healthcare Market Regulation Act relied on insurance companies to be central players in making hospitals compete to provide good medical quality at low cost. However, huge differences emerged between the purchasing and marketing departments of some major insurers. Purchasing departments tried to get the *best value deals* with preferred providers; marketing departments applied a strategy of pursuing contracts with all hospitals to provide *maximum choice* for clients. Purchasing departments tried to live up to the new role of private insurance companies as safeguards of quality of care; marketing departments figured that insurance companies were surely not perceived by their clients as caring for patients' best interests. Marketing departments feared that patients would see them as profit-oriented organizations that would rather save a few euros than provide the best care. Such concerns were fed by national media reporting on, for example, the Netherlands Association of Medical Specialists choosing a collective insurance arrangement that allowed the insured, rather than the insurer, to choose freely where they would receive their medical care. This was seen as an indication that medical professionals themselves did not trust the insurance companies to make such decisions for them, and that they did not trust all their colleagues to deliver high-quality care. Insurers therefore faced the problem that they were seldom perceived as purchasers of quality (Boonen 2009). One purchaser put it this way:

We still have some work to do to improve our image. We're still not perceived as an insurer that is knowledgeable about quality, that knows where to find the best care.

They [the clients] are suspicious too, because if we recommend something it will probably be because it's cheap rather than good.

The resulting marketing strategy might have seriously jeopardized the relevance of business cases for improving care at low cost. Strategic alliances with luxury hotels would be easier to sell as purchased high quality than improved quality through process improvements that resulted in a lower cost, since for the latter it was harder for insured clients to figure out whether the redesigned care was better value or was cheaper because some corners were cut. Consequently, the calculative devices would have to work really well in making such quality gains visible, if not to the individuals insured, then at least to the insurance companies. But did they?

The measurement tools that seemed faithful allies in the case presented above sometimes acted unpredictably. This could have raised questions from team members in hospitals as to whether they were actually working at all. It proved very hard for the hospitals' improvement teams to use the devices we introduced, an issue that became clear in a series of interviews with two sorts of participants: the program managers of each hospital, who were in charge of all projects in their hospital, and the quality managers working on the project to re-design care processes.[11] Those interviews were held after the first year of the project in all eight hospitals in the first tier of Better Faster. Getting teams to start using the measurement instrument turned out to be far from the smoothest episode in the project. Though hospital teams were generally content with our tool for generating data about the care process, using it did not make their jobs less cumbersome. Producing outcomes and charts required immense effort by the staffs of hospital IT departments, quality managers' offices, and the wards and clinics in which the care took place. Apologetic emails from leaders of local improvement teams began to flow in after the deadline had passed for handing over the baseline measurements to me as national project leader. Medical professionals told me they were embarrassed that their IT systems were unable to produce the requested data. Though virtually all of the projects eventually managed to submit their measurements, they often had to make substantial investments of time and other resources to be able to do so. One quality manager put it this way during the interview:

[Generating data] often required manual work, even to the extent of having an intern sitting with a stopwatch in the consulting room. Some things were just tallied. People made lists. It wasn't picked up as a normal part of the primary process.

Another hospital team generated measurements by going through the paper-based patient records retrospectively and then introducing inserts for the later measurements, so that they would not have to go through the entire medical record again to keep track of the trajectory:

> That was a hell of a job, and then you've only covered 20 patients and that then leads to an immense discussion. "I know that patient and there was this and that reason why it took so long." And now the continuous measurement, with the inserts, I just don't find that feasible. It just doesn't work. Period!

Despite all the manual work with files, the results were often far from complete. Many items needed for enacting *trajectories* instead of isolated *events* were not registered, since hospital information systems were still focused on financial administration, and the health system was historically funded largely by a budget based on a limited set of parameters. So while *financially relevant activities* were registered, since these were important for filling the allotted budgets, crucial steps in the care trajectory unaccompanied by billable activities proved impossible to trace. One quality manager stated:

> Your most important measurement is still, when was the diagnosis finalized? And you can't just trace that back anywhere. The most probable moment is when a patient visits the doctor after lots of diagnostics. It makes it really complicated. The only advantage is that the oncologists simply know their patients by name and so you just dig up those files. You can browse through them and in that way measure those results.

It will come as no surprise that hospital program managers were hopeful about ICT plans to reduce this extra work in the future; they simply could not see their employees just generating measurements all day long.

> Now the art is to get measurement embedded in the organization and make it a part of the working process so that it goes a bit better than how we did the baseline measurements. We'll need to automate that. More manual work doesn't make anybody happy. I won't accept our care coordinators walking round the wards just making lists. They should be able to get this data on their screens very easily.

However, the ICT initiatives that some hospitals started also proved demanding:

> Last year we hired someone in Planning & Control who started working on the system to see what we could get out of it. What has to be registered at the point of care if you want to extract data later on? You can generate some things with the system, but for the rest you simply have to dive into the patient records. This person developed some methods to get reasonably reliable figures but these were disputed structurally, because there will always be differences [with other data sets]. The question then becomes: how big can that difference be? What time should we invest in increasing the reliability of data? You just have to find a way in that.

In another hospital, attempts to design "dashboard" screens that allowed care professionals to monitor their redesigned care processes took many months, including hours of ICT consultancy, without delivering any tangible results.

So it seems there were plenty of reasons why the calculative devices could have been seen as *unable* to reconfigure the health care market into value-driven competition. Figures sorely needed to sustain the claim that financially relevant process improvements had been attained were absent, incomplete, or at best generated through huge investments of time, energy, and money. Whether the devices we introduced "worked" seemed highly contestable, and I would not have been surprised if hospitals' improvement teams had fundamentally challenged the very act of measuring all these steps. Whereas many team members were embarrassed by the fact that their ICT systems were unable to produce the requested data, to me this seemed normal in light of empirical analyses of record keeping and secondary uses of information (Garfinkel 1967; van der Lei 1991; Brown and Duguid 2000; Berg and Goorman 1999). More surprising was that neither the relevance of the calculative space nor its workability was challenged. What seemed to make the devices work was that actors flexibly ascribed different levels of validity to them in different settings. Whereas data could be highly contested in a project meeting with medical specialists, nurses, managers, and consultants, those same data seemed to become "harder" when discussed in a project review with the board of directors, and harder still when presented by a board member to a national audience of colleagues or to an insurance company. The messy practices of generating indicators hardly seemed to affect the ability of the devices to connect costs and qualities. This process, which Latour and Woolgar (1979) called "purification," prevented criticism of the measurement tools. Instead such purification allowed higher management to be untroubled by the struggles their teams and ICT departments underwent to generate those indicators. As one hospital program manager put it:

It simply means providing care. What we're doing here is running a business. And we're rapidly improving that. … You've got lots of indicators that you can all start measuring. But the point is of course to get the indicators that give you the quickest overview of how the process is running. … Actually I want to see only the deviations. I'm not really interested in the figures. I want to see if the light is green, red or yellow. How does it look? I want to see the departments' overviews, and I really want people in those departments to become aware that they'll have to work on this. This also applies to our ward managers. They are directly involved in the care process. When I drop by the ward and ask, how many patients are waiting for discharge here? They should be able to say: zero, four, three, like that. Or, on quality, how many patients have pain score x? When I ask people now, they're not aware, they don't know. They're all doing their best, they're all doing a good job, but they are just not working on that, though it's something that can tell you something about how things are really going in the hospital. How many OR cancellations does the hospital have? That's telling for how the process behind it is organized.

The success of reconfiguring the health market despite serious challenges to the credibility of insurance companies and *despite the absence of unambiguously reliable devices* poses a theoretical puzzle that is hard to solve on Callon's terms. And some years later, when I returned to the Atrium Medical Center and studied the developments in one of the leading insurance companies, the puzzle was even more confusing.

Robust Devices, Fragile Markets

On returning to the Atrium Medical Center a few years after the project, I discovered, to my surprise, that information management for pathways had become far more robust. The Atrium Medical Center had decided to invest in dashboards, an indicator system that would let them keep track of the main items in the patient trajectory that were important for managing their delivery of care. During the project to re-design care processes, creating overviews had been a cumbersome process involving extracting data from various modules of the hospitals' registration and information systems, importing them into Excel files, and cleaning up the data extensively. Now, overviews of the number of visits between colonoscopy and surgery, for example, were readily available and were contrasted with the norm for such care set by the improvement team for this care trajectory. (See figure 4.5.)

However, the improved market devices had not made it easier to trigger the interest of insurers to the new quality-improvement initiatives. During negotiations, insurers often did not show the same level of interest that they initially had. The hospital's quality manager put it this way: "It's up to us to bring everything to do with quality to the negotiating table, and they're hardly interested."

Attempting to make insurers aware of their improved processes, the hospital went to some lengths to tout its quality achievements. At times this led to fairly archetypical forms of commodification. Consider this except from an interview with the quality manager:

quality manager: We have to put quality on the agenda. They're not asking for it, so we have to present it. In a few areas, and these are increasing, we know we have something extra to offer, a discerning product, so we put on a big song and dance—always spontaneous, not very structured—but

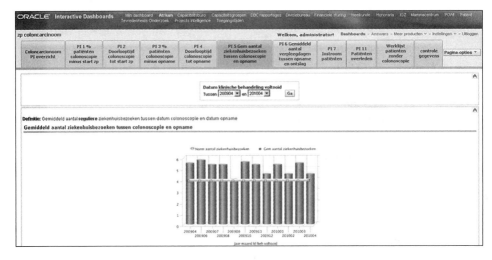

Figure 4.5
Dashboards for quality management: average number of hospital visits between colonoscopy and admission. Courtesy of Atrium MC.

quite a show really, just to make sure the insurer notices. Part of the show involves producing brochures on our discerning care product. We have brochures for our departments of obstetrics, gynecology and pediatrics, nice brochures filled with graphs, protocols and the details various target groups need in the insurance company. We show them off, we say, here, look at this, this is what our care looks like. That's all part of our repertoire.

TZJ: And is it clear to the insurer, that you produce those brochures especially for them?

quality manager: Yes, absolutely. You couldn't give them to anyone else. No patient would think 'this is about me'. They're offered to and discussed explicitly [with the insurer]. Well, and another string on our bow is, of course, that we always get our specialists to join the discussion. So we have two gynecologists talking the medical advisor [of the insurance company] through the process right up to the last injection required after delivery, explaining why that injection really must be included at that moment of this process. In our experience it takes a specialist to convince a medical advisor. But perhaps this model has already lost its force, because now we're seeing that even gynecologists have to sacrifice items in their care products.

Despite having solid process-management indicators, producing sales brochures, and bringing medical specialists into the negotiations to personally specify quality, the hospital found it increasingly hard to sell quality in terms that medical professionals liked to see, even if it were paid for by savings elsewhere in the process.

In economists' discussions about bringing quality into the equation in regulated competition settings, the fact that negotiations sometimes focus more on financial aspects than on medical quality is often explained away by the existence of "information asymmetry." If information on quality is not readily available to all parties, the negotiations will focus on the information that *is* available, and that information tends to be financial, since, as we have seen, financial measures are readily available. Moreover, in the words of Gabriel Tarde, "wealth is something much simpler and more easily measured; for it comprises infinite degrees and very few different types" (1902, as cited in Latour and Lépinay 2009, p. 14). In response to this problem, many actors try to define quality in terms of quality *indicators* with an equal simplicity and transportability that can then be brought into the assessment. A purchaser working for a large insurance company put it this way when I interviewed him about the development of the purchasing process:

What quality indicators could we agree on? This is something we focused on immediately in 2005: we went for that quality. And then we invested a lot, especially in the first years, in discovering what care is actually delivered. That was our input, when we negotiated price, to put actual care delivery next to those quality indicators.

The notion of information asymmetry would suppose that, once transportable performance indicators were available, they would be taken into account in negotiations concerning quality and price. However, the problem emerging in the market for hospital care was that even readily available quality information only became part of the equation in very particular instances, and those instances tend to be instances in which cost saving was an important factor. As the purchaser put it:

If you want to be a preferred provider, then your price has to be below average. It doesn't mean that as soon as someone else goes ten euros cheaper, they get pole position. ... We assume that quality and affordable care can go together. It means that as soon as you [the hospital] do something right but it turns out more expensive, we would be less interested than if it were less expensive.

If quality always came at a lower cost, this statement would not be problematic, but that would be an overly optimistic assumption. Initially all actors in this market thought that substantial gains through changes combining medical quality and cost reduction could be used to make at least some quality investments that would come at a financial cost. Over the years some of the financial gains had been cashed, but the space for making quality investments seemed to evaporate. Contrary to the ideas presented by Callon *and* by health economists, although the information infrastructure for elucidating quality had improved, selling quality had been *easier before*, even though in the early years there had been relatively *poor calculative devices*. The dashboards on quality and cost parameters per care trajectory that had been only managerial dreams in 2007 had actually materialized in recent years. Yet, despite the availability of "valuemeters" that would make actors' value judgments "visible and readable" (Latour and Lépinay 2009, p. 16), it sometimes proved harder to bring quality and cost together in annual negotiations.

In its attempts to still allow for cost-increasing quality improvement that medical professionals deemed necessary, the Atrium Medical Center pursued two strategies: creative bookkeeping (not in the usual pejorative sense) and "playing the patient card." Creative bookkeeping has, of course, become associated with scandals, greed, and the misappropriation of funds. If such normative judgments are left aside, hospitals now literally have more imaginative bookkeeping strategies to ensure the costs incurred for delivering additional quality are actually borne by insurance companies. Such creativity sometimes leads to combining certain treatments into a separate admission, for which a hospital can still charge a different fee. As a division manager explained:

Outpatients with esophagus carcinoma get a PET-CT scan. If deemed necessary after this scan assessment, they also get an endo-echo test on the same day. Because of their illness they are quite frail and so we admit them on day care basis, giving them a bed to recover in between these two big, heavy diagnostic tests. Because of our regional specialization and given the relatively long distances many patients have to travel, day care treatment is all the more important. It's how we reduce hospital visits and manage to create a means of recovering some of our additional costs.

Creative bookkeeping of care products is a strategy that generally does not get much societal acceptance. The literature of health economists refers to it as "upcoding" (Steinbusch et al. 2007), defined as "the practice of miscoding and misclassifying patient data to receive higher reimbursements for services provided" (Lorence and Richards 2002, p. 423)—a practice that health economists see as a "hospital-acquired disease" (Simborg 1981). In a less pejorative sense, it may also be a pragmatic solution, in view of the present complexity of financial streams and the difficulties hospitals face when trying to sell the quality they care about to insurance companies, whose image problem prevents them from simply selling such quality to their insured.

One alternative that would not involve upcoding would be to "play the patient card." In the model of the Dutch market for hospital care, the countervailing power would be individual patients who are expected to change insurers if not satisfied with the way the third-party insurance company looks after their interests (Schut 2009, p. 70). This would encourage the hospital to target patients and their representatives more directly to ensure that insurance companies would be willing to broaden their definition of quality. This is exactly what the Atrium Medical Center is increasingly doing. It has chosen to address citizens and other relevant parties by signing a "contract with society" that includes announcements of highly specific care agreements per diagnosis in local newspapers and in the hospital's quality journal. As the quality manager explains:

It started on our anniversary in 2004, 100 years of Atrium, that was our first contract with society. We used the jubilee year to spend Saturday mornings talking with patient groups in our auditorium and asking general things like, what do we want from each other? The care guarantees [introduced later on] are actually a specification of what started then. Now our contract with society gets adjusted annually and has become far more specific: What do we deliver to our Parkinson's patients? What can [a patient] count on? When is something not good enough? And what penalty card can you hand in where? We've got the support of a management system on our side: are we still delivering what we agreed to deliver?

However, this strategy assumes that insurers will be able to sell better quality at a higher cost to individual clients while excluding some providers from their portfolio of contracted care. Selectively contracting certain hospitals may, however, once again weaken the credibility of insurers. A respondent from the Dutch Healthcare Authority, the government body supposed to regulate and supervise competition on the health care market, stated:

It has to do with the fact that when insurers play hardball in negotiations, they risk not getting a contract. Then they need to explain this to their insured, meaning: you can't go to that hospital any more, or if you do, you will have to pay a substantial part of the cost. This damages reputation and works against the purchase profit.

This explains why insurers increasingly say that quality is quality only if it includes efficiency gains, while hospitals point out that quality not associated with financial advantage is progressively harder to sell. Attempts to improve the quality of care that doesn't fit the insurers' definition have led to strenuous debates between care professionals and managers of hospitals. The professionals are pursuing quality improvement and regional specialization, but evidently that poses a puzzle for hospital managers who, although committed to quality improvement, also have an organization to run.

This was, for example, the case with the development of an esophagus carcinoma trajectory. There was a strong impulse on the national level to centralize treatment of this form of cancer in fewer hospitals, or at least a select number of surgeons to carry out the operations. Clinical evidence showed that patient mortality had a direct inverse relation to the number of resections surgeons carried out annually (Birkmeyer et al. 2003). The Dutch Healthcare Inspectorate turned this finding into a performance indicator that became part of the indicator set in the second pillar of Better Faster, setting ten such operations per surgeon a year as the minimum norm. The professionals at the Atrium Medical Center took up this challenge and informed their regional colleagues that they were specializing in this type of surgery. They would organize a well-run care trajectory for these patients, as they had done for patients with colorectal cancer and for other diagnoses, and they agreed with colleagues in the region that they would refer these patients to the Atrium Medical Center. These surgeons did exactly what any quality-committed health care inspector could have hoped for. They would be saving lives by making this improvement. However, their strategy seemed perfectly opposed to the management strategy emerging simultaneously to deal with current market arrangements. As the quality manager explained:

There is one promising strategy: reducing the products you lose money on. This is what just about everyone on the market is doing. We do it too, but perhaps we're the last ones to start because it goes against our nature so much: we see surgeons cheerfully bringing in their next target, their regional function. We're probably already one of the largest centers in the country [for esophagus carcinoma]. Hooray! We've had no OR mortality since we picked this up two years ago and we didn't start any procedures where, because of progression or metastasis, we couldn't do anything anyway, which indicates careful diagnostics. Well, if that is the measure, then our surgeons are doing a fantastic job. In fact this makes all of us really happy. Now, however, we have a dominant development, where [managerial] divisions certainly are playing a role. "Bleeders and feeders": what is draining [our resources] and how can we get it to stop. Besides zip codes [refusing expensive care for patients who do not live in the vicinity of the hospital] there is a range of options [used to select who gets into treatment]. Now already, the next "bleeder" won't get in. So the next issue like esophagus will be opposed by many [managers] in the hospital. So when some enthusiastic professional says "I can do it! We have a good ICU and I'll get it together on the ward as well, we can do it together! Can I do it?" we'll say "No way!" That's what we'll say. We're already saying it.

On the one hand this is a typical problem that would occur in any budget-driven system with prices set at the national level without differentiating for quality. However, in regulated competition, hospitals hoped to be able to pay for quality improvement that came at a cost by paying it out of the efficiency gains made in the process, and by selling better quality at a higher price. A few years down the line, however, they no longer displayed this enthusiasm. As the division manager put it:

Look what's happening to the prices in the first batch of [care products], it's quite interesting. In the last four to five years these prices have been harmonizing and stabilizing. You can see a national race to the bottom and I expect this to happen with future batches as well. Then you could have a marvelous care program with all kinds of treatment and service activities, but it's uncertain if this would lead to a higher price. So … we end up with a national fixed price. We [hospitals] are not allowed to discuss [price] with other hospitals, because then we'd immediately get the NMA [the Netherlands Competition Authority, another regulatory agency that supervises fair competition and antitrust] breathing down our necks as care providers developing provider power. But those insurers deal with so many hospitals that they know the average price exactly.

This respondent is pointing out that in his opinion the value of cost reduction is built into the present market through a price mechanism that frames quality in a particular way. Consequently, it is harder to sell high quality than to divest expensive care. And the increased robustness of market devices has been unable to change this fragility in the system of regulated competition.

To explore the surprising situation in which better devices led to poorer markets, let me conclude with some reflections on what this experiment with developing health care markets has to offer for social studies of markets. What has situated intervention in the configuration of a health care market taught us about the role of devices in framing markets? What does this imply for the optimism displayed by authors like Callon about the possibility to do markets differently, if only sociologists cared to get involved with the development of calculative technologies?

Economists and Market Devices as the Right Stuff? Historicity, Probability, and the Sociology of Markets

Barry and Slater (2002b, p. 285) quoted Callon as having claimed that "it is impossible to think of markets and their dynamics without taking into account the materiality of markets and the role of technological devices." With colleagues Callon also states that "markets are one form of economic agencement that is marked typically by circulation, pricing and exchange," and that "without devices … these movements that animate markets would be virtually impossible" (Muniesa, Millo, and Callon 2007, p. 4). This claim has certainly been valuable in opening up social studies of markets, and it also relates to the experimental shaping of markets. At times, however, the focus on devices seems to assign an excessive, privileged agential status to material tools and to the economic scientists who construct them.

In a story based on Garcia-Parpet's 1986 study of the transformation of the market for strawberries in the Sologne region of France,[12] Callon (1999, pp. 191–192) produces an actor whose strength seems somewhat exaggerated:

In the construction of the strawberry market, a young counselor of the Regional Chamber of Agriculture played a central part. The remarkable thing is that his action was largely inspired by his training in economics received at university and his knowledge of neoclassical theory. The project, which he managed to launch through his alliances and skills, can be summed up in a single sentence: the construction of a real market on the pure model of perfect competition proposed in economic handbooks. ... [I]t is no coincidence that the economic practices of the strawberry producers of Sologne correspond to those in economic theory. This economic theory served as a frame of reference to create each element of the market.

However seductive this explanation is, we are reminded by critics of ANT (Amsterdamska 1993; Bloor 1999a,b) not to overstate the agential strength of economic scientists, since they are not acting in historic isolation. Indeed, Callon's account fails to situate the counselor in a wider range of practices that may have been crucial to allowing this Sologne strawberry market to emerge.

Similarly, the reconfiguration of health care markets is not an isolated project for interventionist social scientists. By getting involved in the development of market devices, I learned that sentimental attachment to material agency in Science and Technology Studies is as problematic as it was in the late 1980s and the early 1990s. It risks leading to excessive optimism about the malleability of *de novo* market enactments and a reduced sensitivity to the other dimensions that frame market practices. I therefore propose that social studies of markets as well as experiments in situated intervention with the reconfiguration of health care markets need a sensitivity to what Laurent Thévenot has called prevailing "conventions [that are] involved in the collective creation of 'forms of the probable'" (2002, p. 70). Successful reconfigurations may be produced through developing market devices, but are simultaneously influenced by historically shaped "investment in forms" (Thévenot 1984). Thévenot has observed that actor-network theory is less focused on historically produced consequences than on present-day attempts to reconfigure practices:

[T]he notion of network is very compelling because of its power to embrace in its description a potential list of entities which is much broader than the one offered by models of action and practice. But this notion tends to overlook the heterogeneity of links for the benefit of a unified picture of interconnected entities. (2001, p. 408)

The notion of "forms of the probable" tries to attend to this heterogeneity and historical depth of particular investments in forms. This focus on forms of the probable has consequences for what sociologists face during their involvement in the reconfiguration of markets. On the one hand, the story of the construction of health care markets is about the enactment of calculative agents through the construction of "equipment and devices," as Callon (1999, p. 191) suggests. On the other hand, it is a story of how such devices are made to operate in practices shaped by earlier investments in particular market practices.

The enthusiasm that Callon may inspire for the involvement of researchers in social studies of markets in reconfiguring markets should be tempered by an understanding of the dual meaning of such "re-configuration": it entails a process of *configuring* market practices in health care *anew*, drawing together heterogeneous agencies, yet it produces a *repetition of configurations* that were existent in health care competition and health-care-improvement practices owing to the strength of probable market regimes. With this in mind, situated intervention by scholars in social studies of markets should focus not only on developing market devices but also on analyzing which type of market regimes afford such devices. An excessive focus on the malleability of market practices by developing calculative devices, and a lack of sensitivity to prevailing market forms, may lead to disappointing consequences for situated-intervention research on the subject. In that sense, the case of the reconfiguration of health care markets can also warn us against drawing overly optimistic conclusions about the interventionist potential of sociological research to reconfigure health care markets or other markets from price-driven and service-driven to value-driven. Apparently the market regime tends to focus on quality gains that come at a lower price while increasingly setting standard prices at race-to-the-bottom prices. Such price reductions may be based on truly valuable quality improvement, as shown by the cases of colorectal cancer and small elective surgical procedures, but other hospitals have to match this price, which they may well do by shortening length of stay without making the recommended improvements in the quality of the care or by focusing on care that can most easily be sold at a lucrative price. Managing hospitals through "bleeders and feeders" may be more cynical but is certainly far less cumbersome than pathwaying initiatives. Also, although these efficiency gains can initially be used to fund quality improvement that comes at a higher cost, over time prices stabilize at lower levels, without hospitals' being able to sell quality at a higher cost.

In light of the sociological experiment with the Dutch health care market, whether and to what extent researchers in social studies of markets can actively reshape markets *differently*, to produce examples of "successful reconfiguration," as opposed to just accommodating prevailing market regimes, becomes an important question. As a related thought experiment, try to think through what would have been needed to enact the Sologne strawberry market as a market that was *not* in line with neoclassical economics.

Initially, in the case of the Dutch health care market, increasing financial calculability did not exclude other values despite the fragility of the market devices. Quality that medical professionals and patients valued could remain part of the "orders of worth" (Thévenot 2002, p. 61) that defined the focus of competition. With a more historical focus on the "forms of the probable" in the Dutch health care market, one reason for the initial ease of combining different values may well be that Dutch health insurance companies, hospitals, and regulatory bodies historically have all been involved in an entangled plurality of values. Insurance companies have a long albeit marginal history of negotiating both price and quality with hospital directors and doctors. For many years, insurance companies distributed annual "care innovation funds," and did not focus solely on financial outcomes or on devising "innovations" for improving service by, for example, forming alliances with hotels. The fact that multiple, sometimes contradictory regimes are simultaneously present and institutionalized enhanced the chances of reconfiguring regulated competition in the direction of a value-driven health care market, which initially still had space for selling quality improvements that did not come at a lower cost. In such a setting, researchers in social studies of markets and their calculative devices may still find interesting spaces in which to contribute to the configuration of a market regime. Over time, however, this practice of bringing together a plurality of values was unable to hold up, and the health care market shifted toward including other values to the extent that they were defined in terms of financial savings.

As the ambiguities from the developments of the Dutch health care market indicate, there are important conceptual and practical limitations to a theory that ascribes special agential status to economics and its associated devices without also paying attention to the historical investments in forms. As Donald MacKenzie and Yuval Millo state, leaving historical sensitivity out of a study of markets can lead to "quite mistaken conclusions about performativity" (2003, p. 111). My proposal to enhance "Callonistic" studies of the reconfiguration of health care markets with sensitivity to "forms of the probable" aims to overcome the perhaps excessive expectations of opportunities for situated intervention by scholars in social studies of markets who experiment with a radical reshaping of health care markets. This is not quite the same conclusion that Malcolm Ashmore, Michael Mulkay, and Trevor Pinch reached when they studied attempts by health economists to change health care practices in the United Kingdom. "[The health economists'] disappointments and failures," they wrote, "must stand as a warning to us all of the inherent difficulty of using academic social science as a basis for practical assistance to others." (Ashmore et al. 1989, p. 3) As Simon Cole (2009) has argued, continuing a discussion he started some years before with Michael Lynch (Lynch and Cole 2005), cautionary tales of the potential for social sciences intervention should also be treated with caution. Viewed with hindsight, not only did Ashmore and colleagues underestimate the effect health economists were having on the delivery and organization of health care; their conclusion also stopped them explaining *why and how* health economists were able to have such an effect. Focusing both on the production of calculative devices and the market regimes in which they are introduced may prove invaluable for addressing exactly those questions. A historically sensitive approach may be valuable when sociologists, anthropologists, and researchers in social studies of markets actively engage in reconfiguring health care markets. Besides helping them focus on calculative devices, it will also make them sensitive to aspects of previous regimes that may well need to be preserved or cultivated (or be forcefully excluded) to enable those calculative devices to contribute to markets that care for a wider range of values.

Now that I have discussed the potential of situated intervention for sociologically reconfiguring market practices, let me turn to experimental interventions in initiatives to improve patient safety.

5 Sociological Reconfigurations of Patient Safety: Situated Intervention as Multiple Ontologies

Articulating Agendas of (Researching) Patient Safety

Over the last 15 years, activities in the emerging field of quality and safety improvement in health care are resulting in new practices of governing medicine and posing challenges to prevailing notions of what it means to be a good doctor, a good patient, a good manager, or even a good health care system. Health care is not simply a domain in which patients are cured or cared for; it is increasingly seen as a field full of dangers, and hospitals in particular are increasingly seen as risky places.

When the US Institute of Medicine published its report *To Err Is Human: Building a Safer Health System* (Committee on Quality of Health Care in America 2000), the *Wall Street Journal* and the *Washington Post* published front-page articles citing the conclusion that from 44,000 to 98,000 Americans died each year as a consequence, not of the diseases they were being treated for, but of errors that occurred during hospital treatment.[1] Aside from the large numbers, there were shocking individual cases that indicated problems with the health care system. One of these cases was the dreadful death of Betsy Lehman, the *Boston Globe*'s chief medical columnist, who received a massive overdose of experimental chemotherapy during her cancer treatment at one of the most renowned cancer institutes in the United States, the Dana-Farber Cancer Institute in Boston. Her doctor had prescribed "cyclophosphamide dose 4 grams/square meter (of body surface area) over 4 days" (Kenney 2008, p. 6), but whereas that was intended to be the *total dose* that should be administered *over a period of four days*, it was taken by the person administering the medication to signify the *daily dose* of medication *over a four-day period*. After strong reactions to the medication, classified by care professionals as "normal" responses to this form of experimental treatment, Lehman died in the hospital at the age of 39.

Quality and safety in health care are by no means completely new topics in medical sociology. The quality and the safety of care practices are a
longer-standing topic in the sociology of professions, for example. As Donald Light wrote in his critical reading of such authors as Eliot Freidson and
Andrew Abbott:

> To wistfully remember "the Golden Age of Doctoring" (McKinlay 1999) is to forget
> that it was also the age of gold (Rodwin 1993), the age of unjustified large varia-
> tions of hospitalization and surgery caused by autonomy and lack of accountable
> standards (Wennberg and Gittelsohn 1973), the age of large portions of tests, pre-
> scriptions, operations, and hospitalizations judged to be unnecessary by clinical re-
> searchers (Greenberg 1971), the age of medicalizing social problems (Conrad and
> Schneider 1992), the age of irresponsibly fragmented care in the name of "autono-
> my," the age of escalating prices and overcharging to a degree unknown anywhere
> else in the West (Navaro 1976, Waitzkin 1983, White 1991), the age of provider-
> structured insurance that paid for almost any mistake or poor investment anyone
> happened to make, and the age of corporations moving in to reap the no-lose profits
> of such a world by exploiting the profession on its own terms. (Light 2000, p. 202)

In this sense it has long been clear to medical sociologists that quality and
safety in health care should never be assumed. However, the discussion of
countervailing powers that Light presents as a solution to the problem of
professional autonomy excesses implies that quality and safety are lacking
because of the failure of institutional arrangements that should "help the
profession be as trustworthy as it would like to be, but cannot be on its
own" (ibid., p. 212). But while having countervailing powers in place may
suffice to counter-intentional flaws in health care systems, Light does not
address errors and problems in medical practice that stem from more sys-
temic properties.

The quality-improvement and safety-improvement movements that
emerged in response to the problems in the delivery of health care are
involved in a practice that medical sociology, for many decades, assumed
was their monopoly: analyzing and problematizing medical practice in
substantial and increasingly influential ways. Yet this movement is also
involved in the practice in different ways than medical sociologists have
been. What is particularly interesting about the problematization that
comes from agents of health care improvement is that on the one hand
the criticism *comes from within* influential medical institutions like the US
Institute for Healthcare Improvement, and on the other hand it is coupled
to a strong *agenda for change*, including claims to have privileged access to a
set of solutions. This seems to force those who are not quite considered to
belong to the realm of medical practice (for example, medical sociologists,

who problematize health care without having the same kind of ready-made answers to the questions they raise) to re-specify exactly what they are actually doing.

Whereas the idea that health care is an unsafe place is increasingly presented as an empirical reality, the quality-and-safety movement has been highly instrumental in establishing this notion. The *To Err is Human* report was followed by a series of other reports and white papers published by American and European institutions in which advocates of health care improvement redefined health care institutions in two ways. First, these institutions are *unsafe* because of the many human errors that occur in the provision of care. Second, the safety deficiency can be "fixed" because safety can be "built into" these institutions as a non-human property. This definition has proved highly consequential for improvement and research agendas dealing with patient safety in many international health care settings. It has, for example, resulted in additional funding for safety-improvement programs in the United States (Aspden et al. 2004), provided a substantial boost for the importance of incident monitoring systems in Australia (Runciman 2002), led to the development of a safety-management system in the Netherlands that aims to "attack medical errors" (van Geenen 2005), and resulted in a World Health Organization resolution promoting standardization and evidence-based policies for patient safety (Donaldson 2002). These policy initiatives for improving patient safety draw on the notion that a health care system can be *designed for reliability* (Nolan et al. 2004) by deploying incident registration modules, blame-free reporting schemes, root-cause analysis, and other practices (Iedema, Flaboris, et al. 2006; Iedema, Jorm, et al. 2006; Iedema and Rhodes 2006) aimed at "finding the gaps" in the safety net of health care systems.

This focus on health care organizations and on patient-safety practices as system interventions has been conceptualized as the "deficiency model" of patient safety (Mesman 2007). This model has consequences for the role of researchers in studying safety-improvement practices. This role is often described as providing evidence for effective measures to improve the design of systems of care delivery (Grol, Baker, and Moss 2002). The Netherlands Organization for Health Research and Development (ZonMw) has, for example, developed a patient-safety research program that asks scholars to

acquire *applicable knowledge*, insights and experience of safety in the health care sector in various areas, including:

• identifying *tried and tested success factors* to produce a reporting, registration and analysis system that can be applied in various sectors of health care

• *measures* to improve the safety of complex care processes
• *measures* to prevent avoidable damage related to the prescribing and administering/use of medicines. (ZonMw 2008; emphasis added)

With this focus, the research program defines the role of researchers as "finding factors and measures for safety improvement." Such research agendas are emblematic of instrumental definitions of scientific contributions to the problem of patient safety. This narrow definition of 'usefulness' leaves little space for what is arguably the most productive contribution of a sociology of patient safety: the ability to redefine the problem space of patient safety by interrogating categories that are taken for granted by other actors (Hess 2001, p. 239).

Utilitarian definitions of the sociology of patient safety speak directly to the question of how the social sciences should relate to the practices they study. They make it hard for sociology to do what it does best; at the same time, such definitions pose a legitimacy problem for sociologists, who are asked to live up to the promises of realizing "better" systems designs while "all" they may keep producing are complexifying findings rather than clear "answers" (Jensen 2007; Barry et al. 1999; Riley, Hawe, and Shiell 2005). Such findings are bound to be seen as problematic by policy makers when sociology is considered a resource of expertise with which to elucidate the "factors [that] support or hamper safety" (Grol, Baker, and Moss 2002).

An alternative role for the social sciences would be, rather than to provide answers to pre-defined problems of patient-safety policy, to get involved in "the articulation of new agendas" (Jensen 2008, p. 322) for addressing patient safety. That role gives medical sociologists the opportunity to critically engage with prevailing patient-safety agendas and improvement practices without reverting to a distanced critical stance that cuts off all connections to problems of effectiveness in the delivery of care. This approach analyzes which conceptualizations of "effective care" are enacted through different ways of "doing patient safety" in safety-improvement initiatives, and what their consequences are for the care practices in which they are introduced.

In this chapter, I explore the potential for such contributions to patient safety, by focusing on multiple ontologies. Here 'ontologies' does not refer to the philosophical notion of preconceived *assumptions* about what is true in the world and *from which* actors operate; it refers to particular *ways of doing the world* that have specific *consequences* for the action they afford. This pragmatic definition, which can be referred to as ontology in practice (Mol 2002), allows for a study of how multiple, simultaneous ontologies produce different consequences and afford different possibilities for action. It is therefore exactly the analysis of such ontologies in practice and their politics (Mol 1999) in (the study of) patient safety that I explore as an important role for medical sociology and STS.

The notion of ontological politics and the notion of exploring multiple ontologies thereby are certainly related to sensitivities within STS about how worlds are made. On my understanding, they are also distinctly *different* from many other theoretical notions in STS. This is mentioned here because, in a special issue of *Social Studies of Science* on the "turn to ontology" in STS, Steve Woolgar and Javier Lezaun argue that this turn "can be better understood as another attempt to apply its longstanding core slogan—'it could be otherwise'—this time to the realm of the ontological" (2013, p. 322)—a claim they illustrate by placing the ontology-related notion of "enacting" on a "rough continuum" with such classic STS notions as "social shaping" (ibid., p. 324). This slogan has, however, drawn mainly upon "an appeal to principles of historical and cultural relativism—in different times or in different places it could be otherwise" (Woolgar 1991, p. 24), and is consequently often invoked as "it could *have been* otherwise." The temporality of this slogan therefore seems central to many well-known examples in the Social Construction of Technology (SCOT). To illustrate, Wiebe Bijker's work on the development of bicycles and the influence of relevant social groups on the shaping of bicycle design (1995) surely de-essentializes the historical development of "the" bicycle, but never claims that there are different ways of "doing bicycles" going on at the same time, with different consequences. Such a historical-development perspective, however interesting, is not what multiple ontologies are about (nor, of course, does it mean that multiple ontologies would be free from their respective histories). But even exploration of how "it *could be* different" in the present tense, without understanding the difference as related to developments over time, is not the same as articulating that *different versions* of the phenomena under study *are* enacted *at the same time*.

Such differences are worth emphasizing because they also point to *when* it may be interesting to articulate something in terms of multiple ontologies. It mainly seems relevant to articulate multiple ontologies when singularity is presumed, with problematic consequences for the action repertoires that get left out of such singularizations. The question is, therefore, not whether STS does or should "turn to ontology"; rather, the question of multiple ontologies should mainly be seen as a matter of analytic strategy. When is turning to multiple ontologies interesting in terms of the production of STS knowledge? When and how does it allow STS scholars to relate to their fields in more interesting ways? Without such qualifications, "turning to ontology" becomes a strangely realist exercise in showing that "X is really, really, ontologically multiple" while forgetting that, when taking "enactment" seriously, it is a choice for the STS scholar whether to enact a practice or an object as singular, as multiple, as changing over time, or otherwise. Thus, what I call "multiplicity realism" is not merely a sign of the lurking desire to use the latest STS fad and make sure one's work is "hot"; more problematic, it is an indication of lingering contentious realisms within STS.[2]

Working with multiple ontologies by exploring the different ways in which patient safety is done should, therefore, be seen mainly as an experiment to explore how this approach may be productive for reconfiguring contentiously realist research agendas into more explorative scholarship in situated intervention.

Care for Better

To explore this potentiality of multiple ontologies of quality improvement, I draw on empirical material from the evaluation of Care for Better, a national quality-improvement collaborative for the care sectors in the Netherlands, including care for older adults, care for mentally and physically disabled clients, and home care. This quality-improvement collaborative is similar to the Better Faster collaborative I presented in chapter 4 and was part of a strategy at the Ministry of Health to develop such programs for almost all forms of health care in the Netherlands, internationally a unique policy strategy. The Dutch Ministry of Health launched the improvement collaborative in October of 2005, in the wake of recent Dutch and international debates showing great concern for patient safety in the care sectors (cf. Leape et al. 2006).

Quality-improvement collaboratives have drawn increasing attention since the "discovery" of the "quality chasm" by the US Institute of Medicine (Committee on Quality of Health Care in America 2001). Their development was strongly influenced by the Breakthrough Series that the US Institute of Healthcare Improvement initiated in 1995 (Schouten et al. 2008). Such collaboratives bring together multidisciplinary teams from various health care institutions that want to improve a certain aspect of the provision of care within a set time frame (usually somewhere between 6 and 18 months). Each organization creates an improvement team, generally with three to five members, that participates in national conferences of the collaborative. At conferences, teams attend plenary and concurrent sessions and receive coaching from external "experts" on the subject at hand.

In the starting conferences, participating teams typically develop a set of plan-do-study-act (PDSA) cycles that are supposed to guide the implementation of activities in the following action period. At subsequent working conferences, teams share their experiences and "results" with their peers, thereby producing "learning laboratories" (Senge and Scharmer 2001) in which the collaborative aims to stimulate learning in and between settings.

The Care for Better collaborative was a result of various ongoing quality-improvement initiatives in the Netherlands. As a consequence of this legacy, the improvement teams focus on themes defined as six domains of patient safety (decubitus ulcers, fall prevention, sexual abuse, medication safety, aggression and behavioral problems, and eating and drinking) and the domain of patient autonomy and control.

One of the ideas behind the quality-improvement collaborative is that it should lead to shared learning environments that would increase the spread and implementation of "best practices" (Mittman 2004; Kilo 1998), thus conceptualizing the problem of safety in care practices as related to the "implementation problem." Over the years, the problem of "implementation" has become the main concern of the quality-improvement movement. Work in recent decades on the diffusion of innovations by its conceptual founding father, Everett Rogers (1962), has developed a nearly paradigmatic strength in journals such as *Implementation Science*, the *International Journal for Quality in Health Care*, and *BMJ Quality and Safety*. Rogers (1983) defines the diffusion of innovations as "the process by which an innovation is communicated through certain channels over time among the members of a social system."[3] A crucial aspect of this definition is that the innovation is *spread* through organizations over time, in the course of which organizations or individuals may "adopt" or "resist" the innovation. Studying the factors that lead to adopting innovations has become the primary activity of scholars publishing in these journals, who conceptualize "implementation" as a process guided by impeding or supporting factors of change.

Rather than following this conceptualization of safety improvement as dealing with the "implementation" of interventions that address gaps in the safety net, refiguring the problem of patient safety per se may have substantial consequences for the nature of the "implementation problem," which may precisely contribute to sociologically articulating one of the new agendas for issues of patient safety. The implementation problem may prove not to be the empirical reality that the safety movement addresses, but one largely produced through problematic conceptualizations of safety-improvement practices. Sociologically reconfigured problem spaces can help to create ambivalences around existing notions of patient safety that may be crucial for creating new opportunities for situated intervention in quality-improvement collaboratives. Such a potential for social science to contribute to research on patient safety is largely unaddressed or even silenced by prevailing agendas of research policy. Therefore, this chapter also deals with the question of how to practice scholarship in situated intervention in a setting that mainly expects answers in a pre-defined problem space.

In 2006 the Institute of Health Policy and Management began an evaluation study of the Care for Better collaborative. My colleagues and I were aware that both the national funding agency that provided the grant and actors in the collaborative expected our research to help fill the gap in evidence on the effectiveness of quality collaboratives that was articulated in Øvretveit et al. 2002, in Øvretveit and Gustafson 2002, and in Mittman 2004. Such studies claim that there is little evidence of "the effectiveness of quality-improvement collaboratives or specific components that enhance the effectiveness of such collaboratives, and there is hardly any information about their cost effectiveness and sustainability" (Schouten et al. 2008, pp. 1491–1492).

We did not subscribe to the unproblematized notion of "evidence" that has dominated studies in this field, not because the effectiveness of quality improvement and safety improvement would not be a matter of care, but because it seemed worthwhile to turn this notion from a resource for quality-improvement researchers into a topic for social scientists. Without challenging the monolithic notion of evidence intended to generate "further knowledge on the basic components effectiveness, cost effectiveness, and success factors" (Schouten et al. 2008, p. 1491), it seemed unlikely that we would be able to either learn from or contribute anything *sociologically* to the Care for Better collaborative.

"Usefulness" and Multiple Ontologies in the Social Sciences

In line with the trend to claim a need for more engaged scholarly practices, calls for "useful" forms of sociological analysis have made it into the methodological literature on (medical) evaluation research. Instead of critically studying or "merely" assessing the outcomes of health-care-improvement practices, this literature focuses on the development of other forms of assessment, such as "responsive evaluation" (Guba and Lincoln 1992), "action research" (Senge and Scharmer 2001), and "formative evaluation" (Øvretveit 2002). Since these approaches to evaluation are facing a rigid definition of usefulness, it may come as no surprise that they have a particularly bad name in the literature on safety improvement. Consider the entry on action research in the fourth edition of the *Evaluation Thesaurus*:

Action research: 1. A little-known subfield in the social sciences that can be seen as a precursor to evaluation. 2. More commonly, today, the name for research by teachers on classroom or school phenomena. An excellent idea, but one with a very poor track record. (Scriven 1991b, p. 48)

The rise of evidence-based medicine that began in the mid 1980s has brought a scientistic logic to the practice of health care evaluation—a logic that sees evaluation as an exercise performed independent of the interventions under study and that acts as a post hoc allocation machine of success or failure. By this logic, evaluation studies either can provide convincing allocations of effectiveness or must conclude that "evidence is inconclusive." Alternative modes of evaluation therefore have to perform in a realm that defines the role of social scientists in "scientistic" terms. This implies that research is expected to become "useful" in terms of pre-defined strategies for addressing problems of patient safety by adding sociological insights to the factors hampering implementation. As long as the role of the sociology of patient safety is to contribute to solutions that fit pre-defined notions of effectiveness, such research is bound to appear "useless" and to have a "poor track record."

The alternative I explore in this chapter was the starting point in the evaluation study of the Care for Better collaborative. I was interested in articulating what Jensen (2008, p. 322) called "*more and different* features of the healthcare [safety] system than is usually taken into account by critical outsiders or enthusiastic insiders." To keep from getting caught in a power-knowledge nexus that would force me to balance a naive notion of objectivity—referred to by Paul Bate and Glen Robert as "stand back … and watch the bodies pile up on the pavement" (2002, p. 977)—or becoming engrossed in the initiative without being able to challenge its assumptions, I wanted to analyze the way patient safety was *done* in different ways by different actors. In exploring how such an apparently monolithic entity as the notion of "effectiveness" of safety improvement was enacted very differently by various improvement teams, I was hoping to open up notions such as "spread" and "sustainability" that now captured the collaborative in an implementation logic.

Focusing the sociology of patient safety on multiple ontologies, analyzing different ways in which doing patient safety were present in the initiative, and "re-conceiv[ing] both the object(s) of research and the relations between research subjects and objects" (Barry, Born, and Weszkalnys 2008, p. 25) allowed me to explore different problem spaces of patient safety that, in turn, produced new potentials for situated intervention in the collaborative. Since such a reconfiguration of the agenda was not what we had been invited to do, it was by no means a "smooth ride." In the next section, I turn to how I explored these potentials, first focusing on how the safety-improvement collaborative conceived effective improvement.

Unpacking Effectiveness in Medication Safety

The effectiveness of quality-improvement collaboratives is generally defined as "targets realized" and displayed in the quantitative format of measured performance. Typically, about two months after the initial meeting there is a first working conference to familiarize improvement teams with notions that form part of the "grammar" of performance management, such as the distinctions between structure, process, and outcome indicators (Donabedian 2005), the notion of defining Specific, Measurable, Achievable/Ambitious, Relevant and Time-bound (SMART) targets, and the concept of the "run chart" (a spreadsheet showing progress made on pre-defined indicators over time). According to team members of the thematic projects, improvement cannot be separated from this quantitative format. As one member told the participants in a working conference on autonomy in nursing homes, thereby reenacting the need for a numerical definition of effectiveness in quality improvement, "Lord Kelvin said it first, 'If you cannot measure it, you cannot improve it.'"[4]

The participants in the improvement collaborative are enrolled in a specific set of practices that enact performance measurement as the mythological singularized notion of "effectiveness" that has been discussed and critiqued over the last decades in general terms (Porter 1995, 1997, Power 1997, 2004; Kuhn 1977), and particularly in relation to the improvement of quality and safety in health care (May et al. 2006; Tanenbaum 1994, 2005). However, our aim was not to add to the criticism but to explore what particular problems this singularization of "effectiveness" was posing for the thematic improvement teams that wanted to create a challenging and inspiring improvement environment for the attending institutions.

When I compared the idea of a pre-defined and singularized performance target with the different ways in which improvement teams approached patient safety, I noticed continuous goal-shifting practices taking place. Shifting goals may be problematic from the perspective of the singularized performance target and the wish to generate "evidence" for the effectiveness of improvement collaboratives (Schouten et al. 2008), but in the work of the improvement teams it seemed to stem from reflection on the situated issues that good quality-improvement teams try to generate. It turned out that generic indicators, though carrying the promise of coordinating improvement initiatives, often had to be re-specified or even abandoned in order to produce situated and relevant safety improvement. This issue of needing to shift goals came up, for example, in the thematic project on medication safety.

By defining clear outcome measures for this project, the improvement agents responsible for this theme tried to achieve performance measurement and comparability between improvement teams from various care institutions. They formulated four project targets for all the teams:

1. at least 70% of participating wards should achieve a reduction of medication errors by 30% within one year;
2. at least 80% of participating teams should have formulated a written policy on medication safety;
3. 80% of participating teams should have an operating and organizationally secured registration system for medication errors or near misses;
4. 100% of reported near misses or errors should be actively discussed and if possible translated into an improvement initiative. Feedback to the reporting party should be included in the procedure.

Though the targets were clearly compatible with the SMART requirement, at an initial conference it turned out that they did not quite suit the ambivalences and complexities faced by teams exploring new ways of doing medication safety.

When the teams presented their aims, the team from the northern part of the province of North Holland indicated that its improvement target was clearly in line with the generic target set by the program. That team's aim was to achieve "90% reduction of medication errors." Then members of a team from a nursing home in the southwest of Friesland stated that their problem was that they were not working according to protocol: "Our problem is our village-like way of working. Everything is quite small, quite informal and people prefer to arrange things informally, instead of working to rule." They said that their aim was to develop protocols for handling medication and make sure they are rigorously applied. Members of a team from the east of the Netherlands said that they faced a complex problem: they hade all their protocols in place, all according to the national accreditation norms, yet they had impossibly low numbers of reported errors: "We have 70 reported errors a year in a very large organization. There must be a lot more going on than that!" Consequently, their aim was to increase the number of reported errors.

Although the national improvement team had developed a set of targets, one team wanted to meet them, another team wanted to modify them, and yet another team wanted to attain the absolute opposite: an increase of (reported) medication errors. The third team also made me aware that the second team's aim of "making a protocol" did not actually mean that a team was working productively to decrease medication errors. Once protocols are complete, teams may actually have to take further initiatives to increase reported errors. The experience of the third team problematizes an assumption that is often present in improvement programs: the assumption that when you pay attention to a problem domain, the number of reported errors (initially) increases. It may increase, or it may not. Any initiative, therefore, may lead to more or fewer reported errors, and that may be a good sign or a bad one. What seemed to be a "good" indicator, able to coordinate tensions and complexities, dissolves here into a moving target. At the end of the project, each improvement team may well have a highly compelling story about its success—a story based on extremely ambivalent "outcomes."

The afternoon session complicated things further. A speaker from a large institution caring for the physically disabled gave a talk that the conference's organizers had scheduled because they thought it was a particularly "good practice" for dealing with medication errors. The speaker, a member of the institution's board of directors, explained that her institution had given more responsibility to clients for handling their medication for as long as they could do so. Clients have proved to be more reliable in controlling medication than professionals. At her institution, clients were classified according to their level of independence and were given corresponding responsibilities for handling their medication. The speaker claimed this had a positive effect on medication errors. The problem this induced for care workers, however, was that the medication intake had now become largely an issue for the clients themselves, which seriously changed the role of care professionals. As the speaker explained, when clients now ask a care worker to hand them a bottle of pills because they cannot reach it, or to open the bottle for them because they lack strength in their hands, the care workers should do so *without controlling* the medication they are handing out. One of the main problems that the speaker had faced when proposing this change is that this practice is in conflict with the training of care workers who are clearly instructed that—in order to ensure medication safety—*they should never hand out medication without checking it.* So, as she explained, once clients are classified as independent, care workers must stop controlling them. And yet they still have a crucial responsibility in the process of ensuring medication safety: they should continually observe whether clients are still really capable of handling their own medication. The condition of clients who can at first take care of their own medication may deteriorate, in which case the care institution should take over their medication handling. One of the issues that came up at this institution, however, was that it was hard to assess this sliding scale of the classification: if a care worker found a pill on the floor once, he or she should not immediately jump to the conclusion that the client is no longer capable of handling medication autonomously. But the event should also not go unnoticed. Such events should be discussed with the client. If the client indicates that he had happened to drop the pill, hadn't been able to pick it up, and so had replaced it with a new pill, there may be nothing wrong. But if a care worker begins to find pills on the floor more often, then the case worker must re-assess whether the client is still able to handle medication. Such reclassification always requires skillful communication; according to the speaker, reclassification always takes place in cooperation with the client.

Scheduling this presentation as an example of a "good practice" actually problematized the outcome measurements proposed by members of the improvement team, without their realizing it. At the institution in question, "doing medication safety" had changed from "controlling medication behavior and reporting (near) errors" to "reflecting in a professional discretionary space on which errors are problematic, which are permissible, and helping clients realize when the time has come to hand over their responsibilities."

Two ontologies of medication safety emerged at this conference: one of *controlling medication behavior and reporting (near) errors* and one of *reflecting on the question which errors are problematic and which can be allowed to come to safe care*. Such different ontologies resonate with what Sonja Jerak-Zuiderent (2012, p. 732) terms "two modes of patient safety": "reducing uncertainty to prevent possible errors" and "living with uncertainty." Jerak-Zuiderent (ibid., p. 748) states that, whereas in the first mode errors and safety are "antonyms," in the second mode "uncertain safety practices account for errors neither by filling in gaps in knowledge, nor by endlessly improving the implementation of plans. Instead, they require a genuine reappraisal of the conceptualisation of errors in the production of knowledge. This implies that *errors are not by themselves incompatible with safety*, but rather can be *part of safety*."

This success of self-dependence in medication safety is an interesting example of the risk of striving for fully safe systems (Law 2000) based on the first mode of patient safety, and of the importance of accepting particular errors *as part of* doing safety in health care. Similarly, the shifting goals of the care institution, which had all protocols and reporting systems in place but had hardly any reported medication errors, problematized the pre-defined outcome measures. The way this organization wanted to do medication safety would—if successful—lead to an *increase* in reported medication errors.

These multiple ontologies of patient safety render the outcomes of "rigorous" evaluation studies such as those reported by Schouten et al. (2008) highly ambiguous if not meaningless. The notion that a better score equals "evidence" of safety improvement blurs the situations in which such scores may actually be the cause of the marginalization of safety practices that aim at living with uncertainty. Many evaluation studies of improvement collaboratives make a distinction between the outcomes of "objective effectiveness" as patient satisfaction, and patient's functional status, on the one hand, and "subjective effectiveness" such as perceived team effectiveness by team members, on the other (Cohen and Bailey 1997). The former are generally associated with "real" improvement ; the latter is often associated with "participants feeling that they have worked really hard" while displaying skepticism about the "results" of their efforts. To gloss over other ways of doing medication safety through the unrefined concepts of "objective" and "subjective" effectiveness privileges pre-defined "outcomes" and does not analyze how problems and solutions are actually handled in particular care institutions, which would be an important feature of social studies of patient safety. The sociology of patient safety that addresses the complexities of "results" may therefore be better equipped to interact productively with improvement agents and generate potential for situated intervention. Later in this chapter I will discuss how this analysis helped interaction with these actors. But first I will analyze various ways of doing client participation in the improvement collaborative.

Complexifying Agendas for Client Participation in Patient Safety

In safety improvement in health care, as well as in other domains of the quality-improvement movement, there have been strong pleas to involve clients in redesigning care. As we saw in chapter 3, appealing slogans such as "Nothing about me without me" (Ashton and Richards 2003) emphasize that it is a "no-brainer" to involve patients and clients (CrosskeysMedia 2004). These slogans draw on an under-problematized notion of participation and have been highly consequential for the setting up of collaboratives for safety improvement. The Netherlands has no legal obligation to include clients in improvement initiatives, whereas in the United Kingdom, according to section 242(1B) of the NHS Act of 2006, NHS organizations must make arrangements to involve users and improvement teams are required to have a client member. However, one performance target of the Care for Better collaborative was that every team should have a client (or representative) member. When my more quantitatively oriented colleagues in the evaluation team saw the results of the improvement teams' surveys (which showed the different members of such teams), it became apparent that only 25 percent of the teams had succeeded in including clients. During my observations of the national working conferences I noticed that the number of clients who actually participated in these national events was even lower by far. Although it is the overall goal of the autonomy projects to give clients more of a say in determining their quality of life, only 17.6 percent of the improvement teams in projects for homes for the mentally disabled, homes for the physically disabled, and residential care homes had a client as a member of the team.

These findings could easily be taken to indicate that the project's leaders had failed in encouraging the institutions to include clients in their improvement teams, or that client participation simply has to be developed further and once institutions become more familiar with it they will be including clients. However, rather than focus the discussion on more or less client participation, I wanted to explore the various ontologies of client participation present in the collaborative, thinking these might provide a way out of the problematic notion of participation that had I already found troubling during the case at the hematology/oncology ward (as reported in chapter 3).

At one of the working conferences of the thematic project on improving autonomy for the mentally disabled, a client gave a presentation on the client board that she chairs. It is set up as a trust, separate but in a loose liaison with the care institution in which she lives. An attendant employed by the trust supported the client in her presentation. The client and the attendant had carefully prepared the presentation together, and the attendant was "interviewing" the client in front of the audience. Whenever the client was lost for words or did not understand a question, the attendant gently reminded her of the answer they had rehearsed and the client would say "Ah yes, of course" and carry on.

In this inspiring and at times moving presentation, the client explained how the trust had been started. The previous client board of the care institution had been absolutely unworkable for clients. When they were invited to attend a meeting, in preparation they had to work their way through piles of documents that had not been written for them and were hard to understand. The client said that the pace of the meetings was also way too fast. In their own trust, the clients set their own agenda. The board of the institution can suggest items for the agenda but these can simply be ignored. The trust organizes thematic meetings with no more than one topic on the agenda. The members prepare for the meeting by making a short movie about the issue they want to discuss. After the discussion, they come with recommendations to the board. The topics included moving patients to different rooms, shower policy, and the cooking of meals. There had been some commotion about the fact that sometimes clients were moved to another room without their consent when the professionals at the institute thought there were good enough reasons to do so. Clients found this unacceptable, and their recommendations resulted in a new institute policy that prohibits forced moving of clients: clients now have to give their consent. The discussion of shower policy came from questions about the practice of making male and female clients take showers together, separated only by a shower curtain. The members of the client trust deemed this unacceptable, and their recommendation resulted in a policy whereby clients have a right to privacy and segregation of sexes when showering, even though care workers thought this would be inefficient. The third topic had not yet resulted in new policy, but was discussed because of a proposed policy to prohibit clients and staff members from cooking meals together on the wards. As a consequence of to new hygiene regulations, the only place where food can be prepared is in the professional kitchen, by professional cooks—a policy that causes the place these clients live to be reclassified as an "institution" rather than a "home." The clients challenged this reclassification. The client giving the presentation said that she had told the director of the institution "Well, we find that very strange: you are allowed to cook at home!" She was saying that for clients the care home was not an institution that needed to govern clients; it was their home, in which they needed support.

This client-trust seemed to embody a radically different way of doing involvement and empowerment and problematized the notion of "participation." The client said in her presentation: "We are unique: in other places you are allowed to 'participate.'" On the last word, she pulled a disgusted face, drawing quite some laughter from the audience. She indicated that they had had to create their own space, with their own organizational structure and agenda, instead of improving autonomy through participation in existing structures. To get their message across loud and clear, the speaker said that she refuses to speak to the board in their complicated policy language. As an alternative, the trust offers courses to help clients, clients' parents, and attendants to stand up for their rights on their own terms.

This telling, inspiring example shows that including a client in the improvement team may be a form of client empowerment, but more often is a way of doing autonomy that frustrates their involvement in the improvement of their care. I do not conclude from this that client participation should be discouraged, but there seem to be multiple ontologies of client involvement that warrant more reflection than that afforded by the present sentimental and singular focus on "participation" in safety-improvement teams.

Exploring the Potential of Interventionist Evaluation: Refiguring Usefulness

Though conflating evaluation with intervention is generally associated with "confusing roles" of evaluators and executors (Bate and Robert 2002) in the evaluation logic of quality improvement, in this project it had been turned into an explicit aim of the study design. Consider this quotation from the "knowledge translation" section of the project proposal:

There will be regular feedback on the basis of (intermediary) study results to the program leadership (NIZW [now Vilans—the executing body] and ZonMw [the funding and coordinating body]), which will enable making adjustments to the program on the basis of study results … .

The inclusion of such "formative methods" was welcomed and encouraged both in the reviewers' reports from the international scientific committee assessing our proposal and in the final decision letter from the funding body.

However, members of the collaborative did not immediately share our interest in interventionist evaluation. Our formative intention did not prevent the improvement agents from feeling that we were assessing their work in an effective/not-effective paradigm. Our surveys were seen as cumbersome and the ethnographic part of the research, which did not fit the improvement agents' image of scientific work, caused suspicion. The fact that I was attending conferences and constantly making field notes was associated with "auditing" their activities and seeing if things were done "correctly." Improvement agents soon began to refer to me as "the watchman," as I found out during one of the interviews. To explain that budget accounting and seeing if they did things "right" was the least interesting task for an STS researcher, I gave a presentation to the team meeting of all improvement agents to indicate some of the things that I found worth studying. Furthermore, sometimes the presence of researchers at working conferences was not just intimidating to the improvement agents; it was also seen as a risk to achieving the actual improvement aims. This was the case at a conference on the prevention of sexual abuse where the project leader made a real effort to create a safe environment where teams would be able to openly discuss a subject surrounded by strong taboos. The project leader feared that my sudden attendance would jeopardize this safety and would negatively influence the conference. I would be a new face to the group, and some institutions had had traumatic experiences with local press coverage when instances of sexual abuse had been discovered. As a consequence, I was not granted access.

At other times improvement agents were very eager to get feedback, but even then I had to negotiate what our study could contribute. Such negotiations took place during interviews I conducted, during working conferences I observed, and during presentations I gave at meetings of improvement agents. Several improvement agents said they expected us to answer questions about what "good indicators" were for their improvement themes. I was particularly hesitant to take up a role in which I would have to come up with such "answers" in a problem space defined by the improvement agents, and I also felt I really did not know enough about their improvement practices to make any sensible comments. This was a non-expertise that was harder for my colleagues to claim. They were quantitative organizational sociologists who could be expected to know the literature on available indicators. But aside from the question of whether we had enough expertise in (for example) medication safety to define "good indicators," I felt this would not be the most interesting sociological contribution we could make, nor was it clear to me what we would be learning from such an endeavor. I felt more comfortable and confident about configuring my usefulness for the collaborative in terms of articulating how the different ways of *doing* medication safety required different modes of assessment, led to different notions of "effectiveness" and required other measurement practices. Although I was sympathetic toward the improvement agents' need to measure the outcomes of improvement teams (to enable comparisons and learning between sites), I argued that the situatedness of improvement efforts called for constant awareness and flexibility in goal displacement—a practice they might want to foster, rather than to exclude by setting general indicators.

During interviews and presentations, I therefore encouraged improvement agents to spend far more time at the outset of the improvement programs on defining team-specific indicators for teams focusing on different targets in different ways of improving safety. If teams are critically reflecting on the different ways in which "good medication safety" can be done in their situation, the improvement agents should assist them in defining measures that match their goals. In the case of the medication-safety team that wanted to focus on an increase of reported errors, this could, as I suggested, result in related performance targets of more *reported* errors but a *relative decrease* of the amount of *medication* errors. But I also proposed using stories in collaborative safety-improvement practices. Stories travel too and allow for different types of associations and learning than quantitative "outcomes" because they tend to give a better insight into the process of improvement that can be translated more easily to other improvement practices than bare outcomes alone. Though the manager of the collaborative indicated that our attempts to attend closely to stories made our feedback less sharp and more "anecdotal" than he at times wished, the leader of the autonomy project could resonate well with it. The project leader introduced portfolios that allowed teams to articulate their improvement in ways that were not possible in the quantitative format.

The focus on multiple ontologies also proved productive for reconfiguring discussions of management involvement in safety improvement. From the diffusion perspective that was strongly present in the collaborative, the lack of distribution of improvements throughout organizations was seen as problematic. One main reason was thought to be a dire need for "visionary management." The diagnosis of the improvement agents was that managers were focusing merely on efficiency and finances and were not sufficiently involved in, enthusiastic about, or committed to quality improvement to really contribute to spreading and sustaining organizational change. As a result, at the working conferences the improvement teams were encouraged to maintain regular contact with their management through communication campaigns and to keep them informed of their progress.

Our study helped articulate that the issue of management involvement is more productively addressed if it is perceived not as a matter of communication but as a matter of ontology, and that how medication safety is *done* is highly consequential for the ways in which management is *implied*. An approach to medication safety that focuses on increased control by professionals, rigorous adherence to protocols, and investment in automated drug-dispensing equipment offers different potentials for management involvement than doing medication safety as increasing clients' self-reliance. The former demands more staff time for medication handling and investments in automated systems, and the latter offers a potential reduction of time spent on medication management. Managerial values are highly shaped by the situation of increased competition and budget cuts in the Dutch care sectors align more easily with the latter way of doing medication safety than with the former.

Such examples helped bring home the point that the Rogerian focus on diffusion and sustainability does not sufficiently address the notion that the alliance of actors to the improvement initiative should be reflected in the *content* of the interventions: when focusing on organization-wide improvement, the teams should *do different things* and not just *communicate better* what they are doing. I therefore urged improvement agents to critically reflect on the different ways in which themes could be approached and the very different "implementation problems" these approaches produce, rather than continue to spend their time organizing "communication workshops." In the continuation of the improvement collaborative, the improvement agents took up this suggestion and set up new projects that focused on early management involvement in the improvement teams and incorporated the longer-term view on organization-wide change right from the start, rather than isolating such wider change initiatives in "spread" and "sustaining" phases that follow "development." Although the change was based on our evaluation, we cannot claim sole responsibility for it. Nonetheless, I like to think that our constant interaction with the improvement agents contributed to the collaborative improvement initiative.

When discussing client participation with improvement agents I tried to shift the focus from the number of participating clients to the difference between meaningful interactions and "mere participation." I suggested therefore that the improvement teams might want to focus on stimulating forms of involving clients in a more situated way, displaying awareness of the type of clients (e.g., including mentally disabled clients in the autonomy-improvement project team or in the aggression and problem behavior team is probably not appropriate) and of the type of project (participation of clients is perhaps more likely in the eating and drinking project than in a project on the prevention of sexual abuse).

This proposed reconfiguration from client participation as an outcome measure to an analysis of meaningful and situated involvement further indicates that including clients will always require *substantial work* by both clients and members of the improvement team. Simply advocating client participation in improvement teams is not enough. Though improvement agents were largely sympathetic to these ideas, the discussions did not result in new client-engagement practices in the collaborative. Productively involving clients seems to be one of the hardest tasks the collaborative faces as the improvement agents' sentimentality about having client members on all improvement teams is rarely disturbed by the substantial efforts needed to create meaningful participation.

Ontologies of (Studying) Patient Safety

Studying patient safety with a focus on multiple ontologies can provide a productive alternative to the narrow definition of "useful research" that regularly confronts sociologists. Where utilitarian renderings of safety research restrict the role of sociologists to finding factors that hinder improvement and measures to assess it, analyzing multiple ontologies in improvement practices explores the potential of sociologists to productively refigure the problem space of patient safety. A focus on ontologies for such research articulates the "usefulness" of the social sciences in a radically different way than trying to adhere to the "benchmark" of the summative evaluation, preferably with a study design that imitates the "gold standard" of the randomized controlled trial (Schouten et al. 2008)—a design that not just sociologists criticize (Lindenauer 2008).

When the usefulness of the social sciences is limited to finding evidence in pre-defined problem spaces, formative evaluations are no more than attempts to make summative evaluations *more* useful without *re-specifying* what such usefulness entails. In such cases, the social sciences contribute to patient-safety practices to the extent that they "operate on the implicit assumption that research is capable of impacting on practice in useful and beneficial ways if only it cares to try" (Jensen 2007, p. 247). With such a narrow definition of "useful research," doing situated intervention in quality-improvement practices is bound to be stuck with what Michael Scriven (1991) called a "poor track record," at least when compared with summative evaluations that can provide very different kinds of "results."

Just as the practices of the safety-improvement teams need a re-specification of their "results" in the light of the situated problems they are trying to address, so should the "outcomes" of the practices of *studying* patient safety also be re-specified in relation to their goal. Though a focus on multiple ontologies will certainly prove barren in terms of "producing evidence" of the under-problematized "effectiveness" of quality-improvement collaboratives, this focus did prove productive for engendering new potentials for situated intervention in quality-improvement practices. In shifting the aim of the sociology of patient safety from "uncovering barriers to implementation" to "unpacking how patient safety is done and which possibilities and problems this produces," we articulated productive ambivalences of quality improvement. Such ambivalences and reconfigurations of problem spaces are highly "useful" for preventing "implementation problems" that tend to be generated by a diffusion approach to safety improvement. A focus on multiple ontologies of patient safety thereby refigures not merely what it means to study safety-improvement initiatives but also redefines the ways in which such research can be useful for enhancing patient-safety-improvement collaboratives.

These attempts of intervening through evaluation also showed that the role of sociological evaluation researcher comes with specific problems for doing situated intervention. Other actors' sets of epistemological expectations of evaluating quality improvement make more experimental scholarly roles problematic. This may partly be explained by the fact that those responsible for carrying out quality-improvement initiatives are not necessarily eager to receive experimental input from actors who will not be held accountable for the outcome of quality-improvement collaboratives. Another reason is that in evaluation research the sociological mode of knowledge production is bound to stay close to what Chunglin Kwa (2011) calls the hypothetical-analogical style of reasoning. Theorizing about the improvement initiative and suggesting changes to quality-improvement agents affords different opportunities for experimental interventions than the more direct, material, and organizational sociological experiments with quality-improvement practices discussed in the previous chapters. The epistemic expectations of scholarly repertoires of evaluation sociology, may therefore produce somewhat of a fractured ecology (Zuiderent, Winthereik, and Berg 2003) for doing evaluative research experiments on situated intervention. I will now explore further such prerequisites of sociological experiments and the ecology of intervening. I will also return to the question of what situated-intervention research has to offer to debates about the normativity of sociological research practices.

Conclusion: Situated Intervention and the Ethics of Specificity

When the protagonist of J. M. Coetzee's 2003 novel *Elizabeth Costello* is standing in front of "the Gate," the gatekeeper asks her to write up a statement on her beliefs. In her first attempt, she claims a dispensation from the condition to enter, composing this declaration:

I am a writer, a trader in fictions. I maintain beliefs only provisionally: fixed beliefs would stand in my way. I change beliefs as I change my habitation or my clothes, according to my needs. On these grounds—professional, vocational—I request exemption from a rule of which I now hear for the first time, namely that every petitioner at the gate should hold to one or more beliefs.

Not surprisingly, the request isn't granted. The gatekeeper drops the sheet of paper on the floor and hands Elizabeth a new sheet saying "What you believe."

Elizabeth's second attempt is more successful; it gets her past the gatekeeper. But now she must appear before a team of judges and defend her declaration. She claims:

I am a writer, and what I write is what I hear. I am a secretary of the invisible, one of many secretaries over the ages. That is my calling: dictation secretary. It is not for me to interrogate, to judge what is given me. I merely write down the words and test them, test their soundness, to make sure I have heard right. Before I can pass on I am required to state my beliefs. I reply: a good secretary should have no beliefs. It is inappropriate to the function. A secretary should merely be in readiness, waiting for the call. In my work a belief is a resistance, an obstacle. I try to empty myself of resistances.

One of the judges says "Without beliefs we are not human." Elizabeth replies that she is not bereft of all belief. "I have beliefs but I do not believe in them. They are not important enough to believe in. My heart is not in them. My heart and my sense of duty." The judges find these insufficient grounds to grant Elizabeth entrance through the gate, so she has to make a third attempt.

This time Elizabeth claims to believe in what is there, regardless of whether she believes in it or not. She believes in the frogs that appeared in her childhood when the rains came back to Australia. She believes in the river that the frogs live in. "I believe in what does not bother to believe in me." When confronted by a judge with the contradiction in her second declaration, she claims that her present "she" is different than the one "she" was then. Both are real and neither is. "I am an other." When they seem to give up on her, she states "I am not confused." "Yes, you are not confused," one judge replies. "But who is it who is not confused?" The judges begin giggling and then, losing all dignity, burst out in roaring laughter.

Later that day, Elizabeth meets the gatekeeper and tells him that it hadn't gone all that well. She asks if she stands any chance to make it through the gate. He says "We all stand a chance." "But as a writer," she insists, "what kind of a chance do I stand as a writer, with the specific problems of a writer, the specific fidelities?" The gatekeeper says it's not up to him to decide this. But when Elizabeth asks whether he meets many people like her, in her situation, he finally looks up from his work and says "All the time. We see people like you all the time."

Shunning Beliefs, Facing the Charges

The problem that Elizabeth Costello runs into sounds familiar to many social scientists who experimentally intervene in the practices they study. Their stubborn unwillingness to prioritize sentimental beliefs over specific issues in practice gets challenged sometimes by actors who have problems with such ethical flexibility. And at such times it can be hard to convey the importance of acknowledging their normative attachments that previously stood the "test of soundness" while following Howard Becker's advice on preventing sentimentality (1967) and not turning this attachment into something they believe in.

The ethical flexibility that situated intervention cultivates regularly meets sociological judges of all kinds, as it is often mistaken for a "normative deficit" on their behalf. In such discussions, sociologists are told to develop a normative agenda "apart from the interpretation of relevant actors or 'actants'" (Keulartz et al. 2004, p. 12) that is "more compatible with normative standards" (Hamlett 2003, p. 134). Failing to do so can easily lead to serious charges. The sociological evils I have been charged with in various academic forums include doing "just management," being guilty of "disciplining patients," turning sociology into "the handmaiden of neoliberalism," having "gone native" in improvement agendas, and reducing sociology to "normative empiricism." When I tried specifying why certain normative configurations turned out quite unexpectedly in sociological experiments in health care practices, such specifications were often reevaluated in the light of what one of my judges called "Archimedean ethical points" in sociology. From such an ethical vantage point, scholars would hope to be normatively removed from the subject studied and have a comprehensive view of the ethics at stake, similar to the external point from which Archimedes proposed that he could lift the world if given a strong enough lever. As some of these charges came at STS conferences, I have come to find that specificity about normativity gets powerfully challenged at times even in constructivist fields. When extending calls for situatedness and specificity from *scientific knowledge* production to the production of *normativity*, in STS, as in ethical philosophy, "the amoralist, or even his more theoretical associate the relativist, is presented … as an alarming figure, a threat" (Williams 1985, p. 25).

The harshest allegation that scholars of situated intervention may face is that their normative position is depicted as opening the door to Nazism. Star wrote about this in a section of the introduction to *Ecologies of Knowledge* (a section headed, brilliantly, "Why I Am Not a Nazi: Realism and Relativism in Science and Technology Studies"): "It took me a while to figure out what people were talking about in these accusations, since being a Nazi is anathema to me." (1995, p. 11) The reasoning behind this conflation of "relativism, amoralism, and disorder" (Williams 1985, p. 25) is that "fascism requires a kind of situation ethics and requires that one redefine the situation according to opportunism or a kind of distorted view [because of which] any attempt to make relative any situations … becomes morally threatening" (Star 1995, p. 11). The charges of constructivism leading to "flexible fascism" (Fuller 1999, p. 23) have been exacerbated by increasing relations between the state, industry, and universities. According to the zealots of pre-stated normative commitments, such relations are the source of "an aversion to normative judgments and even an open antagonism to the adoption of 'critical' perspectives" (ibid., p. 6), as stronger normative positions would challenge the relationships with research funders. As a further consequence, the scholar who tries to cultivate normative specificity is presented as someone who "refuses to revise, let alone improve, our understanding of the world, but merely holds a mirror to it" (ibid., p. 29). In works by some authors (among them Steve Fuller), within just a few pages one can see constructivism accused of being totalitarian and of being impotent.

The replies to these charges in relation to epistemology have been made convincingly. To quote Star again:

We honestly believe that there are no positions that are epistemologically superior to any others. But I do at the same time argue with and try to overthrow those I don't agree with! Relativism in this sense does *not* imply neutrality—rather, it implies forswearing claims to absolute epistemological authority. This is quite different from abandoning moral commitments. (1995, p. 22)

Similarly, a hesitation to endorse claims about absolute *normative* authority opens up another space for even stronger (because more specifically situated) moral commitments than any Archimedean ethics could offer. A normativity that includes doubt is, in that sense, by no means weaker than more absolutist normativity and, as I have shown throughout this book, offers renewed experimental spaces that could hardly be described as "merely holding up a mirror to practice."

In the empirical chapters of this book, I have tried to present a cogent defense for an attached but unsentimental approach to experiments in the social sciences, thereby turning normativity into an empirical topic in situated-intervention research. Focusing on empirically unpacking specific issues through sociological experiments proved important to a range of health care practices in the projects I was involved in. Shunning belief in non-compliance as a problem of effective delivery of care *as well as* belief in celebrating the complexity of the life-worlds of chronic patients enabled me to articulate *specifically problematic* moments of non-compliance. The combination of patients dealing with scarce medication that required careful handling in order to be effective, the exceptional practice of redistributing unused medication to other patients when coagulation factor concentrates came back from vacation trips, and the somewhat unusual position of hemophilia doctors, regarded as visitors by a steady group of chronic patients, seemed to justify attempts to improve adherence to medication management during vacations. Yet it did not prevent me from creating more space for the complexities of living with hemophilia by installing, or rather formalizing, a nurse-led hemophilia clinic in which such difficulties could be discussed. In this way morbidity and mortality risks could be reduced without unjustifiably marginalizing identities other than that of being a hemophiliac.

Attachments-gone-beliefs also tend to play a substantial role in many of the debates on standardization in health care. In chapter 2 I explored the consequences for hematology and oncology care of bypassing the dichotomous beliefs of universal standardization and unique individualization. Again by focusing on empirically unpacked issues in the delivery of care at this large outpatient clinic and day care treatment center, standardization could be situated in those very issues, which also helped to further articulate them. It contributed to substantial reductions in the time surgery hours ran late and to a better distribution of the workload at the day care treatment center. Thus the tyranny of structurelessness and the fallacy of "one size fits all" (Lampland and Star 2009) could be prevented in favor of empirically specifying what issue which standard tried to address. This also proved relevant for understanding how situated standardization (standardization that is explicitly related to specific issues) differs from the notion of niche standardization (standardization that takes place at the level of the social group), which hopefully helps to move more radically away from the universality/specificity dichotomy that structures virtually all debates on standardization in health care. Thus situated intervention was not merely relevant to the health care practices I was involved in; it also translated sociological theory into other, perhaps relevant concepts.

In the case of situated intervention in creating patient-centered care, an empirical analysis of the organizational changes at the hematology/ oncology outpatient clinic showed how defining patient-centeredness as an attitude of doctors or as the participatory activities of patients could have surprising results and be highly coercive. These notions of patient-centeredness could not preclude that professionals had unparalleled control over their patients, since both fail to acknowledge the complicated relation that these actors are inherently tied up in. A more organizational definition of patient-centeredness helped to focus on exploring the *interrelatedness and dynamics* of issues and interventions: it was only through failing to introduce nurse-practitioners to oncological care trajectories that I learned that sociological attachments to studying invisible *skilled* work at lower hierarchical levels did not match the situation encountered on this ward. The problems I faced when introducing nurse-practitioners helped me to articulate the *lack* of invisible skill and professionalism of nurses who would have had to take up the role of becoming nurse-practitioners. It made me adapt the intervention to introducing more modest nurse-led clinics that were mainly aimed at initiating collaboration between doctors and nurses, and also at generating awareness among nurses of the abilities they lacked, which would prepare the grounds for more substantive re-delegation of tasks in the future. Just as diagnoses and treatments are not neatly separated in distinct phases in medical practice (Berg 1997), the practices of articulating and intervening in issues should be dynamically related to be productive (Schein 1987). Situated standardization is therefore both about relating standards to specific issues and about finding out what the issues are through standardization efforts.

When studying situated intervention in health care markets, I shunned the belief that health care is not a market and the belief that markets produce efficiency and quality in order to explore how market arrangements could be configured so that they would focus on the improvement of a wider range of values, rather than on financial gain alone. Situated intervention in market practices enabled such value-oriented market arrangements, which produced radical changes in the way oncological and surgical trajectories were organized. Throughput time reductions of more than 90 percent for small surgical procedures matched reduced suffering for patients, as they could be served more swiftly and would have to come to the hospital only once. In oncological care trajectories, inconvenient double diagnostic procedures were removed and inpatient days reduced through innovative nutrition and pain-management practices. These improvements also resulted in higher revenue for hospitals, and the market devices that I introduced in the improvement trajectories made visible the cost of poor quality and the potential of quality management as a business strategy. In view of the many problems associated with their use in improvement practices, it was highly surprising, however, that these devices were considered to "work." This posed serious puzzles for the theories within the social studies of markets that ascribed strong agency to such devices for including a wider range of values, but never explained what made such devices work.

Furthermore, the initial changes in oncological and surgical trajectories were still able to accommodate both improvements resulting in financial savings and costly quality investments that could be paid for from the savings. However, it became increasingly hard to sell aspects of quality improvement that did *not* lead to direct increases in monetary value, especially since patients lacked faith in their insurance companies as guardians of quality. This experience thus pointed to the risk of turning STS attachments about the importance of situating agency in market devices into beliefs about where the action is. Such beliefs could easily lead to overly optimistic conclusions about the potential of researchers in social studies of markets to change market arrangements and blind out that they could do so only if their actions matched predominating, historically grown relations.

This chapter thereby showed that sentimentality should be prevented not only in relation to the *societal* attachments of social scientists, but also in relation to their *intellectual* predispositions. Surely an awareness of the importance of *material* interventions is arguably among the most important things that STS has to offer to the wider field of sociologically inspired intervention research. Without stressing this insight, social scientists, even those in STS, tend to revert to purely discursive interventions in material practices, which severely restricts the experimental possibilities for exploring new partial connections and may also strongly reduce the chances of success for social-science interventions. As Hans Harbers concisely put it (2005a, p. 269), "political materials deserve material politics." It is, however, worth remembering that such material politics enter a scene that is already sorted in many ways. Such sorting can result from market practices in other societal domains, including specific notions about the importance of price in market arrangements, about the complexities of professional interests, about the viability of health care providers or insurance companies, and about many other things that historically shape the probable forms an intervention will or will not take. The encountered setting may surely be affected by the interventions, so I am certainly not proposing a return to "context" as the explanation from beyond. Yet, as Kristin Asdal and Ingunn Moser have rightly argued, it is worth noting that STS methods that used to be so sensitive to historical developments have turned to the present to such an extent that a sensitivity to collective practices of "contexting" has largely disappeared from much STS analysis (Asdal and Moser 2012, p. 301). A renewed appreciation of contexting also shows how encountered settings can be highly influential in defining the political potential of the material politics that scholars in social studies of markets propose. This also revives humility about the potential of situated-intervention research to do something that differs radically from the collective contexting that is always already going on. It thereby calls attention to what Michael Lynch calls "topical contextures." As Lynch notes (1991, p. 53), "it would be incorrect to say that any particular application ... *creates* a space of operations; rather, any such application participates in a contexture of activities in which a space is organized." The notion of topical contextures thus provides conceptual machinery for *avoiding the unnecessary hardening of the categories* (Watson-Verran and Turnbull 1995), while remaining equally sensitive to the fact that *precisely such hardening* is being done by many other actors over extended periods of time.

In the case of evaluation as intervention in the Care for Better collaborative, I focused on such topical contextures with the main aim of opening up the dominant image of patient safety such contextures produced. These contextures strongly enacted the belief that "the" problem of patient safety needed to be solved in a pre-defined policy agenda. This resulted in a scholarly role of objectively assessing effective improvement, that, as a dominant image, was so contrary to situated intervention that articulating the ontological multiplicity of "effectiveness" was decisive for opening up space to intervene experimentally in potentially productive ways. Focusing excessively on the ongoing contexting itself and trying to address it critically, may well have precluded an arguably far more "useful" sociological contribution. In this case I therefore decided to take inspiration from Irma van der Ploeg, who noted that "the 'discovery' of contingency and of the deconstructability of so many modernist categories or dichotomies in itself, is not a good reason to make contingency and dissolution of boundaries … into new heroes" (2001, p. 130). As far as I'm concerned, this applies equally to the "discovery" of the importance of historicity, contexting, and topical contextures. Their value for (e.g.) challenging the agency that scholars in the social studies of markets ascribe to market devices does not justify rendering them into conceptual heroes that are to be lent *a priori* credibility.

As a matter of analytic strategy, rather than emphasize the historical elements and topical contextures of quality and safety in health care, I therefore focused on elucidating multiple ontologies of medication safety and client participation. By articulating different ways of improving quality and safety that were not related to historical developments over time but were equally present in the quality-improvement collaborative, I could render visible improvement practices that were made invisible by a narrow patient-safety agenda. Opening up this agenda to ontologically multiple efforts to improve quality and safety allowed me to point to action repertoires that were otherwise overlooked. This proved helpful for overcoming the implementation problems the improvement agents faced, not by finding the "factors" that caused these problems, but by showing how specific improvement agendas in fact created them. But although some members of the Care for Better quality-improvement collaborative appreciated the analytical focus on different ways of improving safety, the management of that program would have preferred outcomes to be less "anecdotal" and kept asking us for more concise, sound data. The experiments with intervening through evaluating thereby indicated that the epistemic expectations actors attach to evaluation research and the fact that sociologists are not directly part of the experimental tinkering seriously limit the opportunities for situated intervention.

This indicates that the approach I explore in this book certainly does not depend on the mere willingness of sociologists to get involved in experimenting and intervening. Given the epistemic and normative expectations by both fellow sociologists and actors in the empirical fields, and given the deflated optimism about the possibilities for devices to change practices in crowded fields with many actors and much contexting going on, situated intervention requires an ecology which provides opportunities for the production of sociological knowledge and located normativities. Without being able to comprehensively describe how such an ecology would look, I will offer a few considerations about the ecologies of intervening.

Ecologies of Situated Intervention

Intervening and the Long Haul

I have discussed individual research projects on situated intervention that are nonetheless intricately interrelated. When I started the project in the hemophilia care center, it seemed challenging but perhaps possible. Some of my initial (and substantial) insecurities about being able to do *anything* in the organization of hospital care with my disciplinary training in the interdiscipline of STS were marvelously soothed at a presentation by a young health care consultant to the staff of a children's hospital on his consultancy's proposal for installing a new electronic medical record. The lack of sensitivity to clinical work, the naive optimism about ICT in health care, and the complete disregard for the experiences of patients and parents of living with a disease did not make me more *sure* of the relevance of my own STS knowledge, but at least it made me aware that having poor knowledge and worse sensitivities was not stopping many others from getting themselves involved in the improvement of health care. I also began to understand that the hesitation of some STS scholars and their criticism—when I was told to better leave such work to professionals—seemed based on a rather naive idea of the expertise of *other* actors involved. My having overcome such initial hesitations in the hemophilia project, and having developed my understanding of health care improvement at least to some extent, later facilitated a project for the larger hematology/oncology ward that the hemophilia care center was part of. In turn, developing the notion and the practices of situated standardization on this ward opened up possibilities for running the pathwaying project on a national level. And without the experience of running an improvement project in a national quality collaborative, the evaluation of Care for Better probably would not have been granted to the research group I belong to, and I would not have been allowed to make the same kind of interventions in that collaborative. Even in these few projects, this shows the importance of institutional history for doing situated intervention. However, such interrelation of experience is obviously not shaped by individual researchers, research teams, or departments merely through long-term involvement (Nowotny 2007).

Refiguring Usefulness through Artful Contamination

In comparing the possibilities for interventionist research in STS and business studies, Steve Brown (2004) notes that STS researchers generally have less of a history of close connections to draw upon and therefore have a harder time than their colleagues in management studies. He also states that, although "scientists and managers are equally involved in the provisional production of order, not least through the deployment of calculative means," "managers seem to need management scholars (for whatever reasons) in a way that scientists do not appear to need STS scholars (perhaps yet)" (ibid., pp. 3–4). The absence of a history of STS intervention is highly influential for the intervention potential, but that may be changing with the rise of many recent intervention practices. Then again, much of the work of management scholars is seen as "needed" precisely because it is not experienced as refiguring the usefulness that managers pre-define—a price that situated-intervention researchers should not be willing to pay for being seen as a resource for the practices studied. The recalcitrance that situated-intervention research cultivates toward agendas set by other actors, and toward normative scholarly attachments, may mean that such research will remain perceived as less univocally useful. And even when it is ascribed value within existing agendas, it may be stubborn enough to still want to change the terms of the perceived usefulness, or it may want to question the attributed usefulness altogether. That STS increasingly *is* seen as potentially useful becomes apparent when Signe Vikkelsø reports on being invited to a meeting with an IT manager of a hospital who said that he was "very interested in doing a 'prospective ANT analysis'" (2007, p. 299)—and this while Vikkelsø was actually more interested in "a more traditional ANT analysis of the [electronic medical record] at work" (ibid.). This observation points to the fact that when actors in hospitals begin to ask for "prospective ANT" it may become harder for STS researchers to legitimize research practices with a different orientation. And an ecology in which intervention starts to become the norm may pose legitimacy problems for other modes of sociological knowledge production as well as for good situated-intervention research itself, since actors in the field begin to define what experimental interventions should be about and contribute to.

Even with such expectations of usefulness, this does not pose immediate problems for doing sociology. STS is a nomadic field—or perhaps a network—with few departments in which STS has internal legitimacy. With all the problems this undoubtedly poses, an interesting consequence is that STS scholars often are perceived as belonging to other disciplinary and institutional settings that are expected to be able to contribute toward practices of engineering, health care, law, environmental issues, business, and management. This has consequences for the ways in which spaces for intervention can be created and are at times ascribed: professionals and policy makers regularly expect intervention to be a logical part of a study when they contract research to the institutes where many STS scholars are based, though they may not necessarily see this as an integral part of knowledge *production*. Yet such institutional settings with their many connections to practices and disciplines often proves consequential for the rhetorical authority STS scholars could claim. In the cases I have discussed in this book, the institute where I worked had many historic and ongoing relations with health care institutions and policy practices, and although claimed rhetorical authority always came with problematic expectations, there was also always space to reconfigure this authority in the experiments that I was involved in. Though I would find it hard to substantiate how to assess whether such flexibility is present in a research project, I do know that when I felt that research agendas were utterly fixed, and usefulness was defined too narrowly, I declined to begin such projects.

If the relations between situated-intervention scholars and their fields are to be productive, I would say that they should be relations of "mutual contamination." Drawing on Chantal Mouffe's conceptualization of contamination (2000, p. 10), this term refers to the idea that sociological attachments and the health care practices under study get entangled in a way that changes in the domain and in the normativity of practice modify the sociologists' identity and their normative concerns—and vice versa. Paraphrasing Lucy Suchman and Randall Trigg's (1991) concept of "artful integration," I propose that situated intervention should be carried out with the aim of achieving *artful contamination*. Contamination is needed on the side of actors in the field to stop sociology from getting locked into pregiven problem spaces that would strongly limit what scholars could offer to their fields. Similarly, contamination is important to prevent sociological attachments from turning into sentimentality, while "anti-bodies" have to be artfully cultivated by being part of strong sociological practices such as continued reading, conference presentations, reviewing papers, and a conducive environment to discuss issues encountered in practice in relation to sociological debates. Artful contamination can be developed by preventing activities of interventionist STS research from becoming sedentary.[1] This is crucial to minimize the risks of cooptation and social engineering (Downey and Lucena 1997).

Partial Connections with Sociology Out There

Requests for prospective actor-network theory analysis also show that the ecologies of sociological intervening are by no means about bringing sociological insights to a sociologically wanting field, and indeed are less and less so. This resonates with what Lynch (2009, p. 108) terms "the surfeit model of PUSS (public understanding of social science)," which implies that social scientists do not offer their fields a sociological conceptualization of their practice, but rather that "the potential recipients of STS wisdom already have at hand their own (occasionally competing) conceptions of what the STS specialist would aim to inform them about" (ibid.). That such surfeits can generate fruitful situations for situated intervention became clear in the project on the hematology/oncology ward when Dr. Palmer, one of the oncologists specialized in palliative care, said that she was particularly interested in the kind of sociology I was doing because she was quite fed up with the medical anthropologists she had encountered in her medical training who had refrained from entering the organizational complexity she was trying to maneuver through every day. She told me:

Then you have someone like Anne-Mei The[2] who comes and tells me that I don't communicate sufficiently and unequivocally with patients about the inevitability of their dying. Well, it's interesting, but it's nothing I'm not already aware of: that's what I'm trying to deal with all the time! But she doesn't tell me what we can do to create the time I would like to have to talk with my patients in a calmer and clearer way!

This was an interesting instance of knowledge translation, since The does more than state that doctors do not spare the time they should take for patients. Her work focuses mainly on instances in which, even when patients and doctors *do* communicate, oncologists can speak enthusiastically of a "good response" to *palliative* treatment, while patients mistakenly but understandably take this as a sign that there may be hope for their survival (The et al. 2000). At the same time Dr. Palmer pointed at an uncomfortable feeling I shared about the absence of organizational complexity in The's analysis, something that is not uncommon in some anthropological analyses that fail to include materiality, organization, and spatial arrangements. Whereas situated standardization aims at the entanglements of organizational specifics and the content of care that is delivered (as I described in chapters 2 and 3), The's focus on communication seems to leave situated organizational arrangements untouched. Dr. Palmer's many insights into (and critical appraisals of) medical anthropology created a connection that proved highly generative when experimenting with introducing nurse-practitioners and re-allocating work from oncologists to these new professionals. She was interested in this experiment because she hoped it would help her overcome her reading of The's diagnosis by generating more time for her to talk to patients without haste and without increasing the burden for her colleagues. Therefore, Dr. Palmer was one of the oncologists most supportive of setting up the nurse-led clinic.

The common denominator of these elements of ecologies of situated intervention is that they largely fall outside the sphere of influence of individual social scientists. An ecological understanding of sociological experiments may therefore serve as both a warning for over-enthusiastic entries into unfavorable settings and a sensitizing concept for exploring the interventionist potential that a specific research site affords. I hope to have shown that when a research setting is conducive for experimental interventions it may provide interesting avenues into a wide range of sociological debates, and into discussions of the normativity of sociology.

An Ethics of Specificity as a Sign of Good Health

To conclude this book, I would like to return to the question of the gains of the approach of situated intervention for the production of scholarly normativity. As I have shown, the gains in terms of improved health care practices have been substantial, though what counted as a gain was often refigured along the way. But this approach has also proved valuable for bypassing the knowledge/power nexus that holds captive much of the sociological debate on the role of scholars in relation to their research domains. Drawing on Casper Bruun Jensen and Peter Lauritsen's (2005) reading of Deleuze 1991, I proposed in the introduction that phrasing the role of the social sciences in relation to their fields in terms of objectivity versus engagement was a "badly posed problem," as it strongly limits the possible intellectual positions of scholars and their imagination about conceivable relations with their fields. Defining social sciences as struggling with a balancing act of detachment and engagement produces what I would like to call a "deficit model of normativity," and draws on the assumption that "real" normativity does not reside in practice and must therefore be created and introduced—perhaps implemented—into practice by social scientists. Practices are seen as facing a deficit of normativity; sociological scholarship may (or should not!) play a role in filling this void.

But just as we have seen an important shift in the public understanding of social science from the "PUSS deficit model" to the "PUSS surfeit model" (Lynch 2009), I propose that situated intervention may be fruitful for shifting the discussion of the sociologists' role toward a model of *normative surfeit* that sociology has to relate to. This reconfigures the sociological challenge from one of adding normative standards to one of dealing with the overflowing normativities encountered in a setting one is involved in. This is obviously not an attempt to enact sociologists as exempt from normative attachments or as merely loyal to local specificity. It is, rather, a

research practice that avoids sentimentality by getting closer to the normative surfeit of practices by getting involved in this surfeit through experimental interventions. The resultant normative-surfeit model of situated
intervention does not seem to need a translation of situated normativities
into beliefs. Rather, it points to the value of an *ethics of specificity*[3] for sociological research.

Such an ethics fruitfully bypasses the knowledge-power nexus, and
thereby addresses some pathological characteristics of the debate on the
role of sociology in relation to its fields of study. Georges Canguilhem—a
medically trained philosopher of science who mainly studied life sciences
and who greatly influenced the work of Michel Foucault—stated in his
groundbreaking work *On the Normal and the Pathological* that although we
usually tend to assume that the pathological involves a departure from the
norm and that ill health is defined as a state of "absence of normality"
(1978, p. 137), this is quite contrary to biological reality (ibid.). Steve Brown
and Paul Stenner powerfully paraphrase Canguilhem's biologically inspired
definition of health:

To be healthy is to be adaptive, to be able to respond to the challenges of the environment flexibly and changeably. This *variability in response is the capacity for normativity*—the ability to become attuned to a range of possible norms. By contrast,
pathology is typically characterised either by a *lack of adaptive responses*, or by becoming *locked into a single response despite changes in conditions*. When interpreted
in this way, health is related to the prior capacity for normativity of the organism,
whilst pathology becomes the reduction of this capacity, for whatever reason, to a
single norm. (2009, p. 160, emphasis added)

Calls for constructivist social sciences to address their "normative deficit" (Keulartz et al. 2004, p. 12) or their "normative vacuum" (Fuller 1999,
p. 27) by adhering to "normative standards" (Hamlett 2003, p. 134) are
generally presented as a remedy for a pathological lack of normativity in
such social sciences. However, the sentimental normativity that sociologists would need to add to the practices they study are unlikely to facilitate a variability in response. Normative standards or Archimedean ethical
points risk becoming a single response and thereby reducing the capacity
for normativity that the authors who prescribed them were claiming to
strengthen. The idea that normativity needs to be added to constructivist
social science distinctly "separates abstract knowledge from practical action
… and implicitly prioritises knowledge over action" (Jerak-Zuiderent 2012,
p. 734), rather than fostering "living with [normative] uncertainty" (ibid.,
p. 735). A normative deficit model therefore prioritizes scholarly representations of normativity, whereas living with an uncertain normative surfeit

situates both the production of sociological knowledge *and* of normativity in the interlocking of representing and intervening (Hacking 1983). Seeing normativity with Canguilhem as the indeterminate surplus of possibilities to respond to a given situation turns the introduction of normative standards into an assault on sociology's *health* in the guise of *normativity*. Canguilhem writes:

Behind all apparent normality, one must look to see if it is capable of tolerating infractions of the norm, of overcoming contradictions, of dealing with conflicts. Any normality open to possible future correction is *authentic normativity, or health*. Any normality limited to maintaining itself, hostile to any variations in the themes that express it, and incapable of adapting to new situations is a normality *devoid of normative intention*. When confronted with any apparently normal situation, it is therefore important to ask whether the norms that it embodies are creative norms, norms with a forward thrust, or, on the contrary, conservative norms, norms whose trust is toward the past (1994, pp. 351–352, emphasis added).[4]

An ethics of specificity for social-science interventions privileges authentic normativity that is adoptive to the setting it encounters over seemingly normative responses that are actually about normality that is devoid of normative intention. A sensitivity to this "ontological difference between the capacity for normativity and the local practices of 'norming'" (Brown and Stenner 2009, p. 160) lies at the heart of situated intervention. It thereby prevents the "harms that result when norms are treated rigidly, and become detached from events, threatening located and lived modes of knowing" (Jerak-Zuiderent 2012, p. 749).

Rather than give in to pathological norming practices, situated intervention articulates a normativity *and* knowledge production that takes its inspiration from the adaptive powers of the biological organism. Within an ethics of specificity, when practices of hemophilia home treatment marginalize doctors rather than patients while non-compliance produces substantial medication-safety risks, sociological attachments to resisting medicalization can surely be adapted. An ethics of specificity equally engenders hesitation about hasty criticism of neoliberalism in health care when one realizes that health economics is trying to develop market devices aimed at articulating public values. And when situated-intervention experiments show that some nurses turn out to be less able and skillful than others, an ethics of specificity allows one to defer commitment to empowering nurses by articulating their invisible work. Situated intervention thus ensures that social scientists are in the good company of patients, doctors, nurses, managers, and all other actors involved in the surfeit of adaptive normativities in health care and other practices. Sociology does not have access to special repositories of normativity, but rather has real lessons to learn from the practices it studies and the ways in which these challenge sociological attachments. Health care practices are full of actors who refuse to turn adaptive normativity into pathological beliefs, and who are able to combine normative attachments with situated practices. This probably applies equally to other fields that sociologists would like to experiment with. After all, the gatekeeper sees people like Elizabeth Costello all the time.

Notes

Introduction

1. Throughout the empirical sections of this book I use pseudonyms that are similar to the original names. I use first or last names according to how people were addressed at meetings.

2. This difference is regarded as crucial to the disciplinary identities of the Germanic and Anglo-Saxon sociological traditions. (See de Wilde 1992.)

3. Many similar studies are discussed in this book. Important studies on improvement of the quality of health care include Bal and Mastboom 2007, Markussen and Olesen 2007, Mesman 2007, and Berg 1998. On workplace ICT design, see Blomberg, Suchman, and Trigg 1996, Knobel and Bowker 2011, and Suchman 2000. On the production of evidence in forensic pathology, see Cole 2001 and Cole 2009. On scientific laboratory work, see Doubleday and Viseu 2007 and Fisher 2007.

4. Quoted on p. 102 of Lynch 2009.

5. See, e.g., Latour 2004.

6. This situation increasingly makes actors direct competitors of funding, with sociologists standing accused of "market contamination"—an issue to which I return in chapter 4.

7. They do not elaborate extensively on this remark, but it seems they are making a point related to the "Mode 2" and "Triple Helix" discussions (Gibbons et al. 1994; Etzkowitz and Leydesdorff 2000), both of which are beyond the scope of this book.

8. For detailed accounts of the diversity in this school, see Fine 1995 and Bulmer 1984.

9. Drawing on the work of Samuel Gilmore (1988), Howard Becker (2008) convincingly argues that this was more of a school of *activity* than a school of thought. Interestingly, Becker pays scant attention to the importance of shared units of analysis for such a school of activity to function, whereas urbanization and other shared

topics such as deviance surely seem relevant in engendering the Second Chicago School.

10. A more moderate version can be found in Galliher 1995.

11. For a more elaborate analysis of the ambiguities in this text and of the problems of a radical reading of Becker, see Hammersley 2001.

12. Hammersley (2001) raises this point in relation to the work of Ned Polsky (1967). Polsky's position is strikingly similar to Becker's, published in the same year, but in a very different style, and has largely gone unnoticed.

13. See Platt 1975 for further iterations.

14. For a similar argument, see Tittle 2004.

15. Of course, it also points to the consequences for the journal one selects to make one's point. Relevantly, Gold reviewed the *Journal of Health and Social Behavior*, whereas Timmermans and Haas reviewed articles from *Sociology of Health and Illness*. Had Timmermans and Haas included the former journal in their analysis, they might have reached a more nuanced notion of the field, and they could have empirically explored the problems of close relations with medicine and the problems of confining sociology to issues of health and illness. See Levine 1987 for a more historical explanation of the different conclusions reached by Gold and by Timmermans and Haas, including an exploration of the concept of "quality of life" that does not impose the choice on sociology to be *in* or *of* medicine but rather proposes sociology *with* medicine.

16. This tension also was observed by Barry et al. (1999), by Jensen (2007), and by Riley, Hawe, and Shiell (2005).

17. This legitimacy issue is, of course, similar to that posed by other adjectives, including "evidence-based" medicine (Guyatt, Cairns, and Churchill 1992), "patient-centered" care (Stewart et al. 1995), and "strong" democracy (Barber 1984).

18. Chunglin Kwa (2011), drawing on the work of Alistair Crombie (2003), calls scientific theorizing "the hypothetical-analogical style of reasoning."

19. Some of the debates—the most vigorous is known as the "science wars"—are firmly beyond the scope of this book, if only because wars don't need repeating.

20. Despite various attempts, I have been unable to find this passage in the work that is generally cited (Lewin 1951), nor have I encountered any citation that specifies a page number. This seems to put it in the company of other famous quotations that are not quite present in the cited work. One such quotation appears in note 4 to chapter 5.

21. For an interesting discussion of this notion (or, rather, of "experimentality"), see www.lancaster.ac.uk/experimentality/. Thanks to Willemine Willems for encouraging me to specify this reading of experimentation.

22. Or Crombie or Kwa, for that matter.

23. Quoted on p. 149 of Lynch 1993.

24. There is, of course, no principled reason why intervention could not also be enacted as a resource. In fact, that is precisely what Chris Argyris does in his work on double-loop learning. "Intervention," he writes (2005, pp. 273–274), "is the most effective methodology for empirical research, related to double-loop learning. Interventions are social experiments where understanding and explanation are in the service of valid implementation intended to be of help." Similarly, there is no principled reason why engagement could not be invoked as a topic, as Casper Bruun Jensen and Peter Lauritsen do (2005, p. 73), and as Saul Halfon and colleagues do in a paper (under review) in which they argue for engagement with agonism rather than engagement as clear and possibly sentimental position taking.

25. The strong emancipatory drive and methodological focus of action research have become all the more visible since the journal *Action Research* published a special issue on *Theory in Action Research* (Dick, Stringer, and Huxham 2009a). Discussing the role of theory without even needing to specify *what* theory shows how foreign this terrain is to this field. Not surprisingly, the question of what "theory" offers to action research is far from answered. According to the conclusions presented in that special issue, although the role of theory in action research is relevant and useful, discussing theory raises more questions than it answers: "It seems that frameworks are useful in making sense of the world. But which frameworks? What do they leave out? How accessible are they to participants? What effect does that have on participation, and in turn on actions? These and other questions about theory may have to wait for other occasions." (Dick, Stringer, and Huxham 2009b, p. 117)

26. It is rather odd that in the whole "captives debate" in STS there is no reference to Becker's work and Gouldner's reply, despite the fact that Becker's analysis of impartiality is quite relevant here, while Gouldner even speaks of the "captivity" of the social sciences.

27. For an almost Weberian attempt to secure neutrality through the separation of the politics and methodology of doing STS, see Collins 1990. For a suitable reply, see Martin, Richards, and Scott 1991.

28. This is not the same as stating that doing STS "has politics." As Collins's contribution to the discussion nicely illustrates, STS researchers tend to claim that things "have politics" without first defining and enacting these things as political in nature. Noortje Marres calls this "a strangely naturalist understanding of politics" (2005, p. 29).

29. Another aspect of this captivity is that sociologists, through their different relations to the various sides of the controversy, also have asymmetrical access to material. Evelleen Richards describes how her attempt at a symmetrical study of the

controversy over using vitamin C for cancer treatment led to supportive access to the personal files of Linus Pauling and colleagues. Meanwhile, the proponents of the other side of the controversy (whom Richards, in far less symmetrical and rather more debunking terms, refers to as "orthodox American oncologists") would not even grant her the time for an interview. She writes that the situation "resulted in a systematic bias in the documentation of the controversy, although this bias is not necessarily to the advantage of the vitamin C advocates. Perhaps its most significant implication is that it lays open to the closest scrutiny the expressed actions, beliefs, and motivations of the supporters of vitamin C, while leaving those of their opponents undeclared except insofar as they are willing to represent them to the other side or in published accounts of their work. The main danger of this situation is that the claims of those most closely scrutinized may be perceived to be 'biased' by the revelation of the supposedly 'nonscientific' factors that have fed into their assumptions, procedures, and presentation of their work, while those of their opponents remain relatively unscrutinized and, perhaps, may be presumed freer of such contaminating influences." (Scott, Richards, and Martin 1990, p. 488) Though the risk of a description of the knowledge production of the underprivileged party may lead to its further loss of status is quite similar to the situation in which the sociologists of deviance found themselves when providing a detailed analysis of groups labeled as deviant, the fact that this situation is produced *through* the very relation to the controversy makes the metaphor of captivity in this respect quite apt. I thank Ingemar Bohlin for pointing this out.

30. Quoted on p. 236 of Hess 2001.

31. An observation that clearly points to the problematic nature of the notion of "going native" in anthropology. This notion immediately forces anthropologists to justify themselves by showing sufficient analytical distance, which closes off so many interesting and relevant ways of relating to our fields.

32. I thank Lise Bitsch for pointing out this risk.

33. See, for example, Winthereik, de Bont, and Berg 2002.

34. Medical coordinators are doctors responsible for managing medical aspects of the work on the ward. They are part of the dual management; the "organizational" part is covered by an operational manager.

35. See also the debate on how to act with a policy practice that is multiple and which changes over time (Webster 2007a; Nowotny 2007; Wynne 2007; Webster 2007b).

Chapter 1

1. For example, Callon and Rabeharisoa (2004), Pasveer (1992), Gomart (2002), Willems (1995), Dodier (1998), Berg (1997), van der Ploeg (2001), and Mol (2002).

2. This change took place only in Western Europe, in North America, and in Australia. In other regions there is not a sufficient supply of coagulation factor concentrates to treat patients in this manner.

3. Cryoprecipitate: a substance with a high concentrate of coagulation factors, obtained by freezing and melting blood plasma.

4. Prophylactic treatment is given to keep the coagulation factor in the blood high enough to prevent bleeds.

5. Though it is beyond the scope of this chapter, it would be interesting to investigate compliance when treatment is situated mainly in the hospital. One would expect that "full compliance" would be equally absent.

6. At the time, this group was called Research on IT in Healthcare practice and Management (RITHM), and it focused on the sociotechnical study of information technology and organizational change in health care. The clinicians approached us because a pharmaceutical company producing coagulation factor concentrates offered to finance research into the changes needed for hemophilia care centers. This fund was labeled by the company as "goodwill money" that would otherwise be spent on flyers.

7. In all the empirical material presented, patients are referred to as "he." This is not a sign of sexism or an artefact of bizarre selection of interviewees. Hemophilia patients are always male; women can only be carriers of the disease.

8. Exactly what over-consumption or under-consumption is is subject to debate, as can be seen by looking at the international discussion of differences in national treatment policies (Steen Carlsson et al. 2003).

9. On a global scale, there is such a shortage of medication that about 80 percent of patients receive no treatment with coagulation factor concentrates or even receive no blood transfusions at all (Mannucci 2003).

10. Though blood products are thoroughly screened to decrease contamination risks, the dangers of spreading unknown or "new" diseases can never be fully precluded. In the 1980s, many patients with hemophilia were infected with HIV. There is a very high rate of hepatitis infections among hemophiliacs, and they faced a higher risk of getting infected with Creutzfeldt-Jakob Disease. This makes patients extremely wary of being exposed to "new" diseases.

11. This is not merely because it is very hard to achieve, or because there is often substantial medical debate on *what* patients should comply with, but also because historically it can be argued that balancing the activities of a care provider prescribing with only "approximate accuracy" and patients complying with "only modest fidelity" has enabled mankind to "survive bleeding, cupping, leeches, mustard plasters, turpentine stupes, and Panalba" (Charney 1975, quoted on p. 134 of Willems

1995). Limited compliance may similarly have saved the lives of hemophilia patients in the 1980s, when HIV-infected blood products were distributed.

12. Translation by the author. Original passage: "patienten *vergeten* hun medicijnen, ze hebben er een misschien onuitgesproken *weerstand* tegen en *denken* dat de *ziekte over* is zo gauw ze er geen last meer van hebben."

13. I thank Peter Harteloh for helping with the analysis of treatment data.

14. The quotations are from patient interviews carried out by Gezieneke Aris, whom I would like to thank for doing this. I translated and edited them slightly for the sake of readability.

15. It is important to emphasize here that *what* this "model patient" is *in* the hemophilia care center is similarly equivocal.

16. Pharmaceutical companies claim on their websites that they have their own fleets of transportation vehicles. Delivering medication in accordance with first-class safety regulations cannot be outsourced; they consider this to be part of their "core competence."

17. I thank David Hess for pointing out these tensions.

18. 'Distance' should be taken here in a metaphorical sense. This is worth mentioning because the physical distance between patients and care centers is a hot topic among the patient association, hemophilia care centers, and the Ministry of Health, which have different ideas about what a good balance would be between the standards a care center should live up to and the need for geographic distribution of centers.

Chapter 2

1. However, those founding fathers were quick to warn against applying such a hierarchy to all clinical questions (Sackett et al. 1996). For a position paper reappraising such early understandings of EBM, see Zuiderent-Jerak, Forland, and Macbeth 2012.

2. See, for example, Grol and Grimshaw 1999 and Roila 2004.

3. An interesting parallel can be drawn here with the study of ICT implementation factors in health care. A study by an international group of medical informatics researchers reported a "total of 110 success factors and 27 failure criteria ... distributed on categories like functional, organizational, behavioral, technical, managerial, political, cultural, legal, strategy, economy, education and user acceptance. ... All success factors and failure criteria were considered relevant by the Delphi expert panel. There is no small set of relevant factors or indicators, but success or failure of a Health ICT depends on a large set of issues." (Bender et al. 2006, p. 125) Though

their conclusion leads them almost to conceptualize the implementation process as a mess, they do not question the usefulness of the study of "factors."

4. ICPs are also known as causal pathways, (coordinated) care pathways, critical (care) pathways, anticipated recovery pathways, and care maps.

5. The European Pathway Association's conference on Care Pathways for Quality Improvement (http://www.healthcareconferencesuk.co.uk/care-pathways-for-quality -improvement) tried to strengthen the understanding of a care pathway as an "individualized tool to support improvement in patient care."

6. Quoted on p. 227 of Epstein 2007.

7. However, as Dan Neyland rightly commented, one may question how long such a position of non-expertise can be maintained once more and more STS researchers have positions in business schools, are involved in ever more practical forms of organizational research, and are called upon to act with other actors in very practical ways. For an interesting exploration of the erosion of the stance of non-expertise, see Vikkelsø 2007.

8. For further elaboration of this approach, see Berg, Schellekens, and Bergen 2005.

9. Although I am sympathetic to work arguing for the power of paper and against the myth of the paperless office (Sellen and Harper 2002), this particular use of paper was nothing to be sentimental about. Nobody missed these overviews when they were no longer part of the paper records.

Chapter 3

1. For classic examples from three decades, see Parsons 1951, Friedson 1960, and Strauss et al. 1997.

2. This distinction is made by Mead and Bower (2000, p. 1088) and by Benzing (2000).

3. Quoted in Mead and Bower 2000.

4. For an interesting analysis of the limitations of patient-satisfaction questionnaires, see Edwards, Staniszweska, and Crichton 2004.

5. I will return to this issue in chapter 5.

6. See Benhabib 1996 and de Wilde 1997.

Chapter 4

1. Broos, CEO of the hospital group, in a press release dated May 2, 2005.

2. For strategic reasons, the Atrium Medical Center requested that I use fictitious numbers. The numbers in this chapter are, however, fairly close to reality.

3. Moreover, as Helen Verran helpfully clarifies, it is important to realize that, though Smith is often referenced as a protagonist of *competition*, this is not quite what he argued. Smith's work needs to be read in the context of the Hobbesian concern of preventing a "war of all against all" (*bellum omnium contra omnes*). This concern, itself much influenced by the English Civil War (1642–1651), made Smith focus on the role of *exchange* as a way of preventing the emergence of such a state. Only the Chicago School (of Economics) focused their interpretation of Smith's main work on *competition* as a key mechanism for preventing Hobbes' much feared and deeply cruel "state of nature." By shifting the focus from exchange to competition, they in fact argued that what was needed was a *fair* war of all against all—a proposal that for both Hobbes and Smith seems anathema (Verran 2012).

4. Referred to in Schut 2003. I thank Erik Schut and Anne-Fleur Roos for their helpful comments on a previous version of this chapter

5. Quoted in Schut 2003.

6. For an empirical analysis of the consequences of these indicators for quality-improvement practices, see Jerak-Zuiderent and Bal 2011. For an analysis of stories on the emergence of these indicators and their relations to what the developers saw as "alter" to their aims, see Jerak-Zuiderent in press.

7. For an optimistic account of the construction of the indicators, see Berg et al. 2005. For a generatively critical reading, see Jerak-Zuiderent in press and Jerak-Zuiderent and Bal 2011.

8. I shared the position with Raymond Sanders of the Netherlands Association of Medical Specialists. I thank him for the collaboration.

9. Marc Berg, Marije Stoffer, and Marc Rouppe van der Voort. I am very grateful for the opportunity to work with them.

10. Our Excel expert was Jeroen Wien from the Dutch Institute for Healthcare Improvement. I'm grateful for his expertise and enthusiasm.

11. I alone conducted all the interviews together with Marije Stoffer, except those at the Atrium Medical Center; those were done by Marc Rouppe van der Voort and Marije Stoffer. I am grateful for their contributions.

12. For a translation of Garcia-Parpet's 1986 paper, see Garcia-Parpet 2007.

Chapter 5

1. For critical readings of this report, see Jensen 2008 and Jerak-Zuiderent 2012.

2. Another such lingering realism is the implicit methodological hierarchy in STS, with ethnographic observations as the hallmark of good scholarly work that is "truly empirical." For a critique of this tendency, see Jerak-Zuiderent in press.

3. Cited on p. 65 of McMaster, Vidgen, and Wastell 1997.

4. Interestingly, this team member's PowerPoint slide featured a corruption of the oft-quoted phrase "If you cannot measure, your knowledge is meager and unsatisfactory." In fact, even this quote, already substantially more nuanced, can't be traced back to the writings of Kelvin. In an extensive search, Thomas Kuhn came no closer than "when you cannot express it in numbers, your knowledge is of a meager and unsatisfactory kind" (1977, p. 178). I thank Gwyn Bevan for pointing out this interesting series of translations.

Conclusion

1. I thank Noortje Marres for pointing this out to me.

2. See The 1999 and The et al. 2000.

3. I thank Casper Bruun Jensen for bringing this concept into our discussions.

4. Cited in on p. 160 of Brown and Stenner 2009.

References

Agency for Healthcare Research and Quality. 2011. National Guideline Clearinghouse, U.S. Department of Health and Human Services (http://www.guideline.gov).

Allen, Davina. 2009. From boundary concept to boundary object: The practice and politics of care pathway development. *Social Science & Medicine* 69: 354–361.

Amsterdamska, Olga. 1993. Surely you are joking, Monsieur Latour! *Science, Technology & Human Values* 15 (4): 495–504.

Argyris, Chris. 2005. Double-loop learning in organizations: A theory of action perspective. In *Great Minds in Management*, ed. Ken G. Smith and Michael A. Hitt. Oxford University Press.

Arrow, Kenneth J. 1963. Uncertainty and the welfare economics of medical care. *American Economic Review* 53 (5): 941–973.

Asdal, Kristin, and Ingunn Moser. 2012. Experiments in context and contexting. *Science, Technology & Human Values* 37 (4): 291–306.

Ashmore, Malcolm. 1989. *The Reflexive Thesis: Wrighting Sociology of Scientific Knowledge*. University of Chicago Press.

Ashmore, Malcolm, Michael Mulkay, and Trevor J. Pinch. 1989. *Health and Efficiency: A Sociology of Health Economics*. Open University Press.

Ashton, Melinda, and Linda Richards. 2003. *Nothing About Me Without Me: A Practical Guide for Avoiding Medical Errors*. Trafford.

Aspden, P., J. M. Corrigan, J. Wolcott, and S. M. Erickson, eds. 2004. *Patient Safety: Achieving a New Standard for Care*. National Academies Press.

Bal, Roland. 1998. Boundary dynamics in Dutch standard setting for occupational chemicals. In *The Politics of Chemical Risk*, ed. Roland Bal and Willem Halffman. Kluwer.

Bal, Roland, and Femke Mastboom. 2007. Engaging with technologies in practice: Travelling the Northwest Passage. *Science as Culture* 16 (3): 253–266.

Barad, Karen. 2007. *Meeting the Universe Halfway: Quantum Physics and the Rntanglement of Matter and Meaning*. Duke University Press.

Barad, Karen. 2011. Erasers and erasures: Pinch's unfortunate "uncertainty principle." *Social Studies of Science* 41 (3): 443–454.

Barber, Benjamin. 1984. *Strong Democracy: Participatory Democracy for a New Age*. University of California Press.

Barry, Andrew, Georgina Born, and Gisa Weszkalnys. 2008. Logics of interdisciplinarity. *Economy and Society* 37 (1): 20–49.

Barry, Andrew, and Don Slater. 2002a. Introduction: The technological economy. *Economy and Society* 31 (2): 175–193.

Barry, Andrew, and Don Slater. 2002b. Technology, politics and the market: An interview with Michel Callon. *Economy and Society* 31 (2): 285–306.

Barry, Christine, Nicky Britten, Nick Barber, Colin Bradley, and Fiona Stevenson. 1999. Using reflexivity to optimize teamwork in qualitative research. *Qualitative Health Research* 9 (1): 26–44.

Bate, Paul, and Glenn Robert. 2002. Studying health care "quality" qualitatively: The dilemmas and tensions between different forms of evaluation research within the U.K. National Health Service. *Qualitative Health Research* 12 (7): 966–981.

Bate, Paul, and Glen Robert. 2007. *Bringing User Experience to Healthcare Improvement: The Concepts, Methods and Practices of Experience-Based Design*. Radcliffe.

Becker, Howard S. 1967. Whose side are we on? *Social Problems* 14 (3): 239–247.

Becker, Howard S. 2008. The Chicago School, So-called. http: //home.earthlink .net/~hsbecker/chicago.html.

Bender, J., E. Ammenwerth, P. Nykänen, and J. Talmon. 2006. Factors influencing success and failure of health informatics systems. *Methods of Information in Medicine* 45 (1): 125–136.

Benhabib, Seyla. 1996. *Democracy and Difference: Contesting the Boundaries of the Political*. Princeton University Press.

Benzing, Jozien. 2000. Bridging the gap: The separate worlds of evidence-based medicine and patient-centered medicine. *Patient Education and Counseling* 39: 17–25.

Berdick, Edward L., and Vicky W. Humphries. 1994. Hospital re-engineers to improve patient care. *Health Care Strategic Management* 12 (11): 13–14.

Berg, Marc. 1997. *Rationalizing Medical Work: Decision-Support Techniques and Medical Practices*. MIT Press.

Berg, Marc. 1998. The politics of technology: On bringing social theory into technological design. *Science, Technology & Human Values* 23 (4): 456–490.

Berg, Marc, and Els Goorman. 1999. The contextual nature of medical information. *International Journal of Medical Informatics* 56: 51–60.

Berg, Marc, Yvonne Meijerink, Marit Gras, Anne Goossensen, Wim Schellekens, Jan Haeck, Marjon Kallewaart, and Herre Kingma. 2005. Feasibility first: Developing public performance indicators on patient safety and clinical effectiveness for Dutch hospitals. *Health Policy* 75 (1): 59–73.

Berg, Marc, Wim Schellekens, and Ce Bergen. 2005. Bridging the quality chasm: Integrating professional and organizational approaches to quality. *International Journal for Quality in Health Care* 17: 75–82.

Berg, Marc, and Stefan Timmermans. 2000. Orders and their others: On the constitution of universalities in medical work. *Configurations* 8: 31–61.

Bijker, W. E. 1995. *Of Bicycles, Bakelites and Bulbs: Towards a Theory of Sociotechnical Change,*. MIT Press.

Birkmeyer, John D., Therese A. Stukel, Andrea E. Siewers, Philip P. Goodney, David E. Wennberg, and F. Lee Lucas. 2003. Surgeon volume and operative mortality in the United States. *New England Journal of Medicine* 349 (22): 2117–2127.

Blomberg, Jeanette, Lucy Suchman, and Randall Trigg. 1996. Reflections on a work-oriented design project. *Human-Computer Interaction* 11: 237–265.

Bloor, David. 1976. *Knowledge and Social Imagery*. Routledge & Kegan Paul.

Bloor, David. 1999a. Anti-Latour. *Studies in History and Philosophy of Science* 30 (1): 81–112.

Bloor, David. 1999b. Reply to Bruno Latour. *Studies in History and Philosophy of Science* 30 (1): 131–136.

Blume, Stuart. 2000. Land of hope and glory: Exploring cochlear implantation in the Netherlands. *Science, Technology & Human Values* 25 (2): 139–166.

Boonen, Lieke. 2009. Consumer Channeling in Health Care: (Im)Possible? PhD dissertation, Erasmus University Rotterdam.

Bowker, Geoffrey C. 2005. *Memory Practices in the Sciences*. MIT Press.

Bowker, Geoffrey C., and Susan Leigh Star. 1999. *Sorting Things Out: Classification and Its Consequences*. MIT Press.

Boyd, Cynthia M., Jonathan Darer, Chad Boult, Linda P. Fried, Lisa Boult, and Albert W. Wu. 2005. Clinical practice guidelines and quality of care for older patients with multiple comorbid diseases: implications for pay for performance. *Journal of the American Medical Association* 294 (6): 716–724.

Brown, John Seely, and Paul Duguid. 2000. *The Social Life of Information*. Harvard Business School Press.

Brown, Steve. 2004. As if Bergson had an MBA. Presented at seminar "Does STS Mean Business," Said Business School, Oxford.

Brown, Steve D., and Paul Stenner. 2009. *Psychology Without Foundations: History, Philosophy and Psychosocial Theory*. SAGE.

Bulmer, Martin. 1984. *The Chicago School of Sociology: Institutionalization, Diversity, and the Rise of Sociological Research*. University of Chicago Press.

Burawoy, Michael. 2005. For public sociology. *American Sociological Review* 70 (1): 4–28.

Burawoy, Michael, William Gamson, Charlotte Ryan, Stephen Pfohl, Diana Vaughan, Charles Derber, and Juliet Schor. 2004. Public sociologies: A symposium from Boston College. *Social Problems* 51 (1): 103–130.

Burstin, Helen R., Alasdair Conn, Gary Setnik, Donald W. Rucker, Paul D. Cleary, Anne C. O'Neil, E. John Orav, Colin M. Sox, and Troyen A. Brennan. 1999. Benchmarking and quality improvement: The Harvard Emergency Department Quality Study. *American Journal of Medicine* 107 (5): 437–449.

Cabana, Michael D., Cynthia S. Rand, Neil R. Powe, Albert W. Wu, Modena H. Wilson, Paul-André C. Abboud, and Haya R. Rubin. 1999. Why don't physicians follow clinical practice guidelines? A framework for improvement. *Journal of the American Medical Association* 282 (15): 1458–1465.

Callon, Michel. 1986. Some elements of a sociology of translation: Domestication of the scallops and the fishermen of St. Brieuc Bay. In *Power, Action and Belief: A New Sociology of Knowledge?* ed. John Law. Routledge and Kegan Paul.

Callon, Michel. 1998a. An essay on framing and overflowing: Economic externalities revisited by sociology. In *The Laws of the Markets*, ed. Michel Callon. Blackwell.

Callon, Michel. 1998b. Introduction: The embeddedness of economic markets in economics. In *The Laws of the Markets*, ed. Michel Callon. Blackwell.

Callon, Michel. 1998c. *The Laws of the Markets*. Blackwell.

Callon, Michel. 1999. Actor-network theory: The market test. In *Actor Network Theory and After*, ed. John Law and John Hassard. Blackwell.

Callon, Michel. 2004. Europe wrestling with technology. *Economy and Society* 33 (1): 121–134.

Callon, Michel, Pierre Lascoumes, and Yannick Barthe. 2009. *Acting in an Uncertain World: An Essay on Technical Democracy*. MIT Press.

Callon, Michel, and John Law. 1995. Agency and the Hybrid Collectif. *South Atlantic Quarterly* 94: 481–507.

Callon, Michel, Cécile Méadel, and Vololona Rabeharisoa. 2002. The economy of qualities. *Economy and Society* 31 (2): 194–217.

Callon, Michel, Yuval Millo, and Fabian Muniesa. 2007. *Market Devices*. Blackwell.

Callon, Michel, and Fabian Muniesa. 2005. Economic markets as calculative collective devices. *Organization Studies* 28 (8): 1229–1250.

Callon, Michel, and Vololona Rabeharisoa. 2004. Gino's lesson on humanity: Genetics, mutual entanglements and the sociologist's role. *Economy and Society* 33 (1): 1–27.

Cambrosio, Alberto, and Camille Limoges. 1991. Controversies as governing processes in technology assessment. *Technology Analysis and Strategic Management* 3 (4): 377–396.

Campbell, Harry, Rona Hotchkiss, Nicola Bradshaw, and Mary Porteous. 1998. Integrated care pathways. *British Medical Journal* 316: 133–137.

Canguilhem, Georges. 1978. *On the Normal and the Pathological*. Reidel.

Canguilhem, Georges. 1994. Normality and normativity. In *A Vital Rationalist: Selected Writings from Georges Canguilhem*, ed. François Delaporte. Zone Books.

Cardillo, Alessio, Salvatore Scellato, Vito Latora, and Sergio Porta. 2006. Structural properties of planar graphs of urban street patterns. *Physical Review E* 73 (066107): 1–8.

Cefkin, Melissa. 2009. *Ethnography and the Corporate Encounter: Reflections on Research in and of Corporations*. Berghahn.

Charney, E. 1975. Compliance and prescribance. *American Journal of Diseases of Children* 129: 1009–1010.

Chase, Richard B., and David A. Tansik. 1983. The customer contact model for organization design. *Management Science* 29 (9): 1037–1050.

Chen, Pauline W. 2011. Finding the patient in a sea of guidelines. *New York Times*, May 19.

Clark, Adele, and Susan Leigh Star. 2008. The social worlds framework: A theory/ methods package. In *The Handbook of Science and Technology Studies*, third edition, ed. Edward J. Hackett, Olga Amsterdamska, Michael Lynch, and Judy Wajcman. MIT Press.

Clawson, Dan, Robert Zussman, Joya Misra, Naomi Gerstel, Randall Stokes, Douglas L. Anderton, and Michael Burawoy, eds. 2007. *Public Sociology: Fifteen Eminent Sociologists Debate the Politics and the Profession in the Twenty-First Century*. University of California Press.

Coetzee, J. M. 2003. *Elizabeth Costello: Eight Lessons*. Secker & Warburg.

Cohen, S. G., and D. E. Bailey. 1997. What makes teams work: Group effectiveness research from the shop floor to the executive suite. *Journal of Management* 23: 239–290.

Cole, Simon. 2001. *Suspect Identities: A History of Fingerprinting and Criminal Identification*. Harvard University Press.

Cole, Simon A. 2009. A cautionary tale about cautionary tales about intervention. *Organization* 16 (1): 121–141.

Collins, Harry. 1990. Captives and victims: Comments on Scott Richards and Martin. *Science, Technology & Human Values* 16: 249–251.

Collins, Patricia Hill. 1986. Learning from the outsider within: The sociological significance of black feminist thought. *Social Problems* 33 (6): S14–S32.

Collins, Patricia Hill. 1999. Reflections on the outsider within. *Journal of Career Development* 26 (1): 85–88.

Committee on Quality of Health Care in America. 2000. *To Err Is Human: Building a Safer Health System*. National Academies Press.

Committee on Quality of Health Care in America. 2001. *Crossing the Quality Chasm: A New Health System for the 21st Century*. National Academies Press.

Conein, Bernard, Nicolas Dodier, and Laurent Thevenot. 1993. Les objects dans l'action: De la maison au laboratoire. École des Hautes Études en Sciences Sociales.

Conrad, Peter. 1985. The meaning of medication: Another look at compliance. *Social Science & Medicine* 20 (1): 29–37.

Conrad, Peter. 1987. The noncompliant patient in search of autonomy. *Hastings Center Report* 17 (4): 15–17.

Conrad, Peter, and Joseph W. Schneider. 1992. *Deviance and Medicalization: From Badness to Sickness*. Temple University Press.

CrosskeysMedia. 2004. Involving patients in redesigning care. In *Pursuing Perfection in Health Care* (video series). Institute for Healthcare Improvement.

Deleuze, Gilles. 1991. *Bergsonism*. Zone Books.

Denzin, Norman K. 1968. On the ethics of disguised observation. *Social Problems* 15 (4): 502–504.

Dewey, John. 1929. *The Quest for Certainty: A Study of the Relation of Knowledge and Action*. Minton, Balch.

de Wilde, Rein. 1992. *Discipline en Legende: De identiteit van de sociologie in Duitsland en de Verenigde Staten 1970–1930*. Van Gennep.

de Wilde, Rein. 1997. Sublime futures: Reflections on the modern faith in the compatibility of cummunity, democracy, and technology. In *Technology and Democracy: Obstacles to Democratization*, ed. Sissel Myklebust. Centre for Technology and Culture.

Dick, Bob, Ernie Stringer, and Chris Huxham. 2009a. Theory in action research. *Action Research* 7 (1): 5–12.

Dick, Bob, Ernie Stringer, and Chris Huxham. 2009b. Final reflections, unanswered questions. *Action Research* 7 (1): 117–120.

Dilts, David M. 2005. Practice variation: The Achilles' heel in quality cancer care. *Journal of Clinical Oncology* 23 (25): 5881–5882.

Dodier, Nicolas. 1998. Clinical practice and procedures in occupational medicine: A study of the framing of individuals. In *Differences in Medicine*, ed. Marc Berg and Annemarie Mol. Duke University Press.

Donabedian, Avedis. 2005. Evaluating the quality of medical care. *Milbank Quarterly* 83 (4): 691–729.

Donaldson, Liam. 2002. Championing patient safety: Going global. *Quality & Safety in Health Care* 11: 112.

Doubleday, Robert, and Ana Viseu. 2007. Questioning interdisciplinarity: What roles for laboratory based social science? In *Nano Meets Macro: Social Perspectives on Nanoscale Sciences and Technologies*, ed. Kamilla Lein Kjølberg and Fern Wickson. Pan Stanford.

Downey, Gary Lee, and Joseph Dumit. 1997. Locating and Intervening: An introduction. In *Cyborgs and Citadels: Anthropological Interventions in Emerging Sciences and Technologies*, ed. Gary Lee Downey and Joseph Dumit. School of American Research Press.

Downey, Gary Lee, and Juan C. Lucena. 1997. Engineering selves. In *Cyborgs and Citadels: Anthropological Interventions in Emerging Sciences and Technologies*, ed. Gary Lee Downey and Joseph Dumit. School of American Research Press.

Dy, Sydney M., Pushkal Garg, Dorothy Nyberg, Patricia B. Dawson, Peter J. Pronovost, Laura Morlock, Haya R. Rubin, and Albert W. Wu. 2005. Critical pathway effectiveness: Assessing the impact of patient, hospital care, and pathway characteristics using qualitative comparative analysis. *Health Services Research* 40 (2): 499–516.

Dy, Sydney M., Pushkal Garg, Dorothy Nyberg, Patricia B. Dawson, Peter J. Pronovost, Laura Morlock, Haya R. Rubin, Marie Diener-West, and Albert W. Wu. 2003. Are critical pathways effective for reducing postoperative length of stay? *Medical Care* 41 (5): 637–648.

Eddy, David M., Joshua Adler, Bradley Patterson, Don Lucas, Kurt A. Smith, and Morris Macdonald. 2011. Individualized guidelines: The potential for increasing quality and reducing costs. *Annals of Internal Medicine* 154 (9): 627–634.

Edwards, Carol, Sophie Staniszweska, and Nicola Crichton. 2004. Investigation of the ways in which patients' reports of their satisfaction with healthcare are constructed. *Sociology of Health & Illness* 26 (2): 159–183.

Engeström, Yrjö. 1990. Organized forgetting: An activity-theoretical perspective. In *Learning, Working and Imagining: Twelve Studies in Activity Theory*, ed. Yrjö Engeström. KirjapainoOma Kyssa.

Enthoven, Alain C. 1988. *Theory and Practice of Managed Competition in Healthcare Finance*. Elsevier.

Enthoven, Alain C., and Wynand P. M. M. van de Ven. 2007. Going Dutch: Managed-competition health insurance in the Netherlands. *New England Journal of Medicine* 357 (24): 2421–2423.

Epstein, Steve. 2007. *Inclusion: The Politics of Difference in Medical Research*. University of Chicago Press.

Etzkowitz, Henry, and Loet Leydesdorff. 2000. The dynamics of innovation: From national systems and "Mode 2" to a triple helix of university-industry-government relations. *Research Policy* 29: 109–123.

Evans, J. G. 1995. Evidence-based and evidence-biased medicine. *Age and Ageing* 24: 461–463.

Evans, J. H. III, Y. Hwang, and N. J. Nagarajan. 1997. Cost reduction and process reengineering in hospitals. *Journal of Cost Management*, May/June: 20–27.

Evidence-Based Medicine Working Group. 1992. Evidence-based medicine: A new approach to teaching the practice of medicine. *Journal of the American Medical Association* 268 (17): 2420–2425.c

Faulkner, Alex. 2002. Casing the Joint: The material development of artificial hips. In *Artificial Parts, Practical Lives: Modern Histories of Prosthetics*, ed. Katherine Ott and Stephen Mihm. NYU Press.

Fearong, K. C. H., O. Ljungqvist, M. Von Muyenfeldt, A. Revhaug, C. H. C. Dejong, K. Lassen, J. Nygren, et al. 2005. Enhanced recovery after surgery: A consensus review of clinical care for patients undergoing colonic resection. *Clinical Nutrition* 24 (3): 466–477.

Field, M. J., and K. N. Lohr. 1990. *Clinical Practice Guidelines: Directions for a New Program*. National Academies Press.

Fine, Gary Alan. 1995. *A Second Chicago School? The Development of a Postwar American Sociology*. University of Chicago Press.

Fish, Stanley. 2004. Why we built the ivory tower. *New York Times*, May 21.

Fisher, Erik. 2007. Ethnographic invention: Probing the capacity of laboratory decisions. *NanoEthics* 1 (2): 155–165.

Fisher, Erik. 2011. Public science and technology scholars: Engaging whom? *Science and Engineering Ethics* 17 (4): 607–620.

Ford, Robert C., and Myron D. Fottler. 2000. Creating customer-focused health care organizations. *Health Care Management Review* 25 (4): 18–33.

Freeman, A. C., and K. Sweeney. 2001. Why general practitioners do not implement evidence: Qualitative study. *British Medical Journal* 323: 1100–1105.

Freeman, Howard E., Sol Levine, and Leo G. Reeder. 1963, 1972, 1979. Present status of medical sociology. In *Handbook of Medical Sociology*, first, second, and third editions, ed. Howard E. Freeman, Sol Levine, and Leo G. Reeder. Prentice-Hall.

Friedson, E. 1960. Client control and medical practice. *American Journal of Sociology* 65: 374–382.

Fuller, Steve. 1999. Why science studies has never been critical of science: Some recent lessons on how to be a helpful nuisance and a harmless radical. *Philosophy of the Social Sciences* 30 (1): 5–32.

Galliher, John F. 1995. Chicago's two worlds of deviance research: Whose side are they on? In *A Second Chicago School? The Development of a Postwar American Sociology*, ed. Gary Alan Fine. University of Chicago Press.

Garcia, Marie-France. 1986. La construction sociale d'un marché parfait: le marché au cadran de Fontaines-en-Sologne. *Actes de la Recherche en Sciences Sociales* 65: 2–13.

Garcia-Parpet, Marie-France. 2007. The social construction of a perfect market: The strawberry auction at Fontaines-en-Solonge. In *Do Economists Make Markets? On the Performativity of Economics*, ed. Donald MacKenzie, Fabian Muniesa, and Lucia Siu. Princeton University Press

Garfinkel, Harold. 1967. "Good" organizational reasons for "bad" clinic records. In Garfinkel, *Studies in Ethnomethodology*. Prentice-Hall.

Garfinkel, Harold. 2002. *Ethnomethodology's Program: Working Out Durkheim's Aphorism*. Rowman & Littlefield.

Garfinkel, Harold, and Harvey Sacks. 1970. On formal structures of practical action. In *Theoretical Sociology*, ed. John C. McKinney and Edward A. Teryakian. Appleton-Century-Crofts.

Gibbons, Michael, Camille Limoges, Helga Nowotny, Simon Schwartzman, Peter Scott, and Martin Trow. 1994. *The New Production of Knowledge: The Dynamics of Science and Research in Contemporary Societies*. SAGE.

Gilmore, Samuel. 1988. Schools of activity and innovation. *Sociological Quarterly* 29: 203–219.

Godlee, Fiona. 2006. Say no to the market. *British Medical Journal* 333.

Gold, Margaret. 1977. A crisis of identity: The case of medical sociology. *Journal of Health and Social Behavior* 18 (2): 160–168.

Goldenberg, Maya J. 2006. On evidence and evidence-based medicine: Lessons from the philosophy of science. *Social Science & Medicine* 62 (11): 2621–2632.

Goldstein, M. K., R. W. Coleman, S. W. Tu, R. D. Shankar, M. J. O'Connor, M. A. Musen, S. B. Martins, et al. 2004. Translating research into practice: Organizational issues in implementing automated decision support for hypertension in three medical centers. *Journal of the American Medical Association* 11 (5): 368–376.

Gomart, Emilie. 2002. Methadone: Six effects in search of a substance. *Social Studies of Science* 32 (1): 93–135.

Gouldner, Alvin W. 1968. The sociologist as partisan: Sociology and the welfare state. *American Sociologist* 3 (may): 103–116.

Gray, Denis Pereira. 2005. Evidence-based medicine and patient-centred medicine: The need to harmonize. *Journal of Health Services Research & Policy* 10 (2): 66–68.

Greenberg, Selig. 1971. *The Quality of Mercy: A Report on the Critical Condition of Hospital and Medical Care in America.* Atheneum.

Grilli, Roberto, and Jonathan Lomas. 1994. Evaluating the message: The relationship between compliance rate and the subject of a practice guideline. *Medical Care* 32 (3): 202–213.

Grit, Kor, and Wilfred Dolfsma. 2002. The dynamics of the Dutch health care system: A discourse analysis. *Review of Social Economy* 60 (3): 377–401.

Grol, R. 2000. Implementation of evidence and guidelines in clinical practice: A new field of research? *International Journal for Quality in Health Care* 12 (6): 455–456.

Grol, R., R. Baker, and F. Moss. 2002. Quality improvement research: Understanding the science of change in health care. *Quality & Safety in Health Care* 11 (2): 110–111.

Grol, R., and J. Grimshaw. 1999. Evidence-based implementation of evidence-based medicine. *Joint Commission Journal on Quality Improvement* 25 (10): 503–513.

Grol, R., and M. Wensing. 2004. What drives change? Barriers to and incentives for achieving evidence-based practice. *Medical Journal of Australia* 15 (180): 57–60.

Grol, R., A. Zwaard, H. Mokkink, J. Dalhuijsen, and A. Casparie. 1998. Dissemination of guidelines: Which sources do physicians use in order to be informed? *International Journal for Quality in Health Care* 10 (2): 135–140.

Guba, Egon G., and Yvonna S. Lincoln. 1992. *Effective Evaluation: Improving the Usefulness of Evaluation Results through Responsive and Naturalistic Approaches.* Jossey-Bass.

Guthman, Julie, and Melanie DuPuis. 2006. Embodying neoliberalism: Economy, culture, and the politics of fat. *Environment and Planning D* 24 (3): 427–448.

Guyatt, G., J. Cairns, and D. Churchill. 1992. Evidence-based medicine: A new approach to teaching the practice of medicine. *Journal of the American Medical Association* 268 (17): 2420–2425.

Hacking, Ian. 1983. *Representing and Intervening: Introductory topics in the Philosophy of Natural Science.* Cambridge University Press.

Halffman, Willem. 2003. Boundaries of Regulatory Science: Eco/toxicology and the regulation of aquatic hazards of chemicals in the US, England, and the Netherlands, 1970-1995. PhD dissertation, University of Amsterdam.

Halfon, Saul, Cora Olson, Ann Kilkelly, and Jane Lehr. Under review. TWISTS as theory and practice. *Science as Culture.*

Hamlett, Patrick W. 2003. Technology theory and deliberative democracy. *Science, Technology & Human Values* 28 (1): 112–140.

Hammersley, Martyn. 2001. Which side was Becker on? Questioning political and epistemological radicalism. *Qualitative Research* 1 (1): 91–110.

Haraway, Donna J. 1991a. *Simians, Cyborgs and Women: The Reinvention of Nature.* Routledge.

Haraway, Donna J. 1991b. Situated knowledges: The science question in feminism and the privilege of partial perspective. In *Simians, Cyborgs and Women: The Reinvention of Nature*, ed. Donna J. Haraway. Routledge.

Haraway, Donna J. 1997. *Modest_Witness@Second_Millenium.FemaleMan_Meets_OncoMouse: Feminism and Technoscience.* Routledge.

Harbers, Hans. 2005a. Epilogue: Political materials—material politics. In *Inside the Politics of Technology: Agency and Normativity in the Co-production of Technology and Society*, ed. Hans Harbers. Amsterdam University Press.

Harbers, Hans. 2005b. *Inside the Politics of Technology: Agency and Normativity in the Co-production of Technology and Society.* Amsterdam University Press.

Hedgecoe, Adam. 2004. *The Politics of Personalized Medicine: Pharmacogenetics in the Clinic.* Cambridge University Press.

Helgesson, Claes-Frederik. 2010. From dirty data to credible scientific evidence: Some practices used to clean data in large randomised clinical trials. In *Medical*

Proofs, Social Experiments: Clinical Trials in Shifting Contexts, ed. Catherine Will and Tiago Moreira. Ashgate.

Hess, David. 1997. If you're thinking of living in STS: A guide for the perplexed. In *Cyborgs and Citadels: Anthropological Interventions in Emerging Sciences and Technologies*, ed. Gary Lee Downey and Joseph Dumit. School of American Research Press.

Hess, David. 2001. Ethnography and the development of science and technology studies. In *Handbook of Ethnography*, ed. Paul Atkinson, Amanda Coffey, Sara Delamont, Lyn Lofland, and John Lofland. SAGE.

Iedema, Rick, Arthas Flabouris, Susan Grant, and Christine Jorm. 2006. Narrativizing errors of care: Critical incident reporting in clinical practice. *Social Science & Medicine* 62: 134–144.

Iedema, Rick, Christine Jorm, Debby Long, Jeffrey Braithwaite, Jo Travaglia, and Mary Westbrook. 2006. Turning the medical gaze upon itself: Root cause analysis and the investigation of clinical error. *Social Science & Medicine* 62: 1605–1615.

Iedema, Rick, and Carl Rhodes. 2006. Surveillance, resistance, observance: Exploring the teleo-affective volatility of workplace interaction. *Organization Studies* 27 (8): 1111–1130.

Iscoe, Neill A., Vivek Goel, Keyi Wu, Gord Fehringer, Eric Holowaty, and David Naylor. 1994. Variation in breast cancer surgery in Ontario. *CMAJ: Canadian Medical Association Journal* 150 (3): 345–352.

Jensen, Casper Bruun. 2007. Sorting attachments: On intervention and usefulness in STS and health policy. *Science as Culture* 16 (3): 237–251.

Jensen, Casper Bruun. 2008. Sociology, systems and (patient) safety: Knowledge translations in healthcare policy. *Sociology of Health & Illness* 30 (2): 309–324.

Jensen, Casper Bruun, and Peter Lauritsen. 2005. Qualitative research as partial connection: Bypassing the power-knowledge nexus. *Qualitative Research* 5 (1): 59–77.

Jerak-Zuiderent, Sonja. 2012. Certain uncertainties: Modes of patient safety in healthcare. *Social Studies of Science* 42 (5): 733–753.

Jerak-Zuiderent, Sonja. 2013. Generative Accountability: Comparing with Care. PhD dissertation, Erasmus University Rotterdam.

Jerak-Zuiderent, Sonja. In press. "Keeping open" by re-imagining fears and laughter. *Sociological Review*. DOI: 10.1111/1467-954X.12221.

Jerak-Zuiderent, Sonja, and Roland Bal. 2011. Locating the worths of performance indicators: Performing transparencies and accountabilities in health care. In *The Mutual Construction of Statistics and Society*, ed. Ann Rudinow Sætnan, Heidi Mork Lomell, and Svein Hammer. Routledge.

Jones, Peter. 1984. *Living with Haemophilia*, second edition. MTP.

Kember, Sarah. 2002. Reinventing cyberfeminism: Cyberfeminism and the new biology. *Economy and Society* 31 (4): 626–641.

Kember, Sarah. 2003. *Cyberfeminism and Artificial Life*. Routledge.

Kenney, Charles. 2008. *The Best Practice: How the New Quality Movement Is Transforming Medicine*. Public Affairs.

Keulartz, Josef, Maartje Schermer, Michiel Korthals, and Tsjalling Swierstra. 2004. Ethics in technological culture: A programmatic proposal for a pragmatist approach. *Science, Technology & Human Values* 29 (1): 3–29.

Kilo, Charles M. 1998. A framework for collaborative improvement: Lessons from the Institute for Healthcare Improvement's Breakthrough Series. *Quality Management in Health Care* 6 (4): 1–13.

Kitchiner, Denise, and Peter Bundred. 1998. Integrated care pathways increase use of guidelines. *British Medical Journal* 317: 147.

Knaapen, Loes, Hervé Cazeneuve, Alberto Cambrosio, Patrick Castel, and Beatrice Fervers. 2010. Pragmatic evidence and textual arrangements: A case study of French clinical cancer guidelines. *Social Science & Medicine* 71 (4): 685–692.

Knobel, Cory, and Geoffrey C. Bowker. 2011. Values in design. *Communications of the ACM* 54 (7): 26–28.

Kuhn, Thomas S. 1977. The function of measurement in modern physical science. In *The Essential Tension: Selected Studies in Scientific Tradition and Change*, ed. Thomas S. Kuhn. University of Chicago Press.

Kwa, Chunglin. 2011. *Styles of Knowing: A New History of Science from Ancient Times to the Present*. University of Pittsburgh Press.

Lampland, Martha, and Susan Leigh Star. 2009. *Standards and Their Stories: How Quantifying, Classifying, and Formalizing Practices Shape Everyday Life*. Cornell University Press.

Latour, Bruno. 1987. *Science in Action: How to Follow Scientists and Engineers through Society*. Harvard University Press.

Latour, Bruno. 1988a. Mixing humans and nonhumans together: The sociology of a door-closer. *Social Problems* 35 (3): 298–310.

Latour, Bruno. 1988b. The politics of explanation. In *Knowledge and Reflexivity*, ed. Steve Woolgar. SAGE.

Latour, Bruno. 1990. Drawing things together. In *Representation in Scientific Practice*, ed. Michael Lynch and Steve Woolgar. MIT Press.

Latour, Bruno. 1996. On Actor-Network Theory: A few clarifications. *Soziale Welt* 47 (4): 367–381.

Latour, Bruno. 2004. Why has critique run out of steam? From matters of fact to matters of concern. *Critical Inquiry* 30: 225–248.

Latour, Bruno, and Vincent Antonin Lépinay. 2009. *The Science of Passionate Interests: An Introduction to Gabriel Tarde's Economic Anthropology*. Prickly Paradigm Press.

Latour, Bruno, and Steve Woolgar. 1979. *Laboratory Life: The Construction of Scientific Facts*. SAGE (1986 edition: Princeton University Press).

Law, John. 2000. Ladbroke Grove, or How to Think about Failing Systems. Centre for Science Studies, Lancaster University (http: //www.lancs.ac.uk/fass/sociology/papers/law-ladbroke-grove-failing-systems.pdf).

Law, John. 2004. *After Method: Mess in Social Science Research*. Routledge.

Law, John, and John Urry. 2004. Enacting the social. *Economy and Society* 33 (3): 390–410.

Lawson, Annette. 1991. Whose side are we on now? Ethical issues in social research and medical practice. *Social Science & Medicine* 32 (5): 591–599.

Leape, Lucian L., G. Rogers, D. Hanna, P. Griswold, F. Federico, C. A. Fenn, D. W. Bates, L. Kirle, and B. R. Clarridge. 2006. Developing and implementing new safe practices: Voluntary adoption through statewide collaboratives. *Quality & Safety in Health Care* 15: 289–295.

Leatherman, Sheila, Donald M. Berwick, Debra Iles, Lawrence S Lewin, Frank Davidoff, Thomas Nolan, and Maureen Bisognano. 2003. The business case for quality: Case studies and an analysis. *Health Affairs* 22 (2): 17–30.

Levine, Sol. 1987. The changing terrains in medical sociology: Emergent concern with quality of life. *Journal of Health and Social Behavior* 28 (1): 1–6.

Lewin, Kurt. 1951. *Field Theory in Social Science: Selected Theoretical Papers*. Harper and Row.

Leydesdorff, Loet, and Janelle Ward. 2005. Science shops: A kaleidoscope of science-society collaborations in Europe. *Public Understanding of Science* 14 (4): 353–372.

Light, Donald W. 2000. The medical profession and organizational change: From professional dominance to countervailing power. In *Handbook of Medical Sociology*, ed. Chloe E. Bird, Peter Conrad, and Allen M. Fremont. Prentice-Hall.

Lindenauer, Peter K. 2008. Effects of quality improvement collaboratives are difficult to measure using traditional biomedical research methods. *British Medical Journal* 336: 1448–1449.

Lorence, P., and M. Richards. 2002. Variation in coding influence across the USA: Risk and reward in reimbursement optimization. *Journal of Management in Medicine* 166: 422–435.

Luff, Paul, Jon Hindmarsh, and Christian Heath. 2000. *Workplace Studies: Recovering Work Practice and Informing System Design*. Cambridge University Press.

Lutfey, Karen. 2005. On practices of "good doctoring": Reconsidering the relationship between provider roles and patient adherence. *Sociology of Health & Illness* 27 (4): 421–477.

Lutfey, Karen, and William Wishner. 1999. Beyond "compliance" is "adherence": Improving the prospect of diabetes care. *Diabetes Care* 22 (4): 635–639.

Lynch, Michael. 1991. Laboratory space and the technological complex: An investigation of topical contextures. *Science in Context* 4 (1): 51–78.

Lynch, Michael. 1993. *Scientific Practice and Ordinary Action: Ethomethodology and Social Studies of Science*. Cambridge University Press.

Lynch, Michael. 2006. From ruse to farce. *Social Studies of Science* 36 (6): 819–826.

Lynch, Michael. 2009. Science as a vacation: Deficits, surfeits, PUSS, and doing your own job. *Organization* 16 (1): 101–119.

Lynch, Michael, and Simon Cole. 2005. Science and Technology Studies on trial: Dilemmas of expertise. *Social Studies of Science* 35 (2): 269–311.

MacKenzie, Donald, and Yuval Millo. 2003. Constructing a market, performing theory: The historical sociology of a financial derivatives exchange. *American Journal of Sociology* 109 (1): 107–145.

MacKenzie, Donald, Fabian Muniesa, and Lucia Siu. 2007. *Do Economists Make Markets? On the Performativity of Economics*. Princeton University Press.

Manna, Radjesh, Paul Steinbusch, Joost Zuurbier, and Marc Berg. 2006. Businesscase voor kwaliteit: Kostenbeheersing door maximale inzet op verbetering van zorg. Department of Health, Policy and Management, Erasmus University Rotterdam.

Mannucci, P. M. 2003. Hemophilia: Treatment options in the twenty-first century. *Journal of Thrombosis and Haemostasis* 1 (7): 1349–1355.

Markussen, Randi. 1996. Politics of intervention in design: Feminist reflections on the scandinavian tradition. *AI & Society* 10: 127–141.

Markussen, Randi, and Finn Olesen. 2007. Rhetorical authority in STS-studies of information technology: Reflections on a study of implementation of IT at a hospital ward. *Science as Culture* 16 (3): 267–279.

Marres, Noortje. 2005. *No Issue, No Public: Democratic Deficits after the Displacement of Politics*. University of Amsterdam.

Marrie, Thomas J., Catherine Y. Lau, Susan L. Wheeler, Cindy J. Wong, Margaret K. Vandervoort, and Brian G. Feagan. 2000. A controlled trial of a critical pathway for treatment of community-acquired pneumonia. *Journal of the American Medical Association* 283 (6): 749–755.

Martin, Brian. 1993. The critique of science becomes academic. *Science, Technology & Human Values* 18 (2): 247–259.

Martin, Brian. 1996. Sticking a needle into science: The case of polio vaccines and the origin of AIDS. *Social Studies of Science* 26: 245–276.

Martin, Brian, Evelleen Richards, and Pam Scott. 1991. Who's a captive? Who's a victim? Response to Collins's method talk. *Science, Technology & Human Values* 16 (2): 252–255.

Marx, Karl. 1845. Theses on Feuerbach. In *Marx and Engels: Basic Writings on Politics and Philosophy*, ed. Lewis S. Feuder. Doubleday Anchor.

Massey, Douglas S. 2007. The strength of weak politics. In *Public Sociology: Fifteen Eminent Sociologists Debate the Politics and the Profession in the Twenty-First Century*, ed. Dan Clawson, Robert Zussman, Joya Misra, Naomi Gerstel, Randall Stokes, Douglas L. Anderton, and Michael Burawoy. University of California Press.

May, Carl, Tim Rapley, Tiago Moreira, Tracy Finch, and Ben Heaven. 2006. Techno-governance: Evidence, subjectivity, and the clinical encounter in primary care medicine. *Social Science & Medicine* 62: 1022–1030.

McDonald, Heather, Amit Garg, and Brian Haynes. 2002. Interventions to enhance patient adherence to medication prescriptions. *Journal of the American Medical Association* 288 (22): 2868–2879.

McKinlay, John B. 1999. The end of the golden age of doctoring. *New England Research Institutes Network* 1 (summer): 3.

McMaster, T., R. T. Vidgen, and D. G. Wastell. 1997. Technology transfer: Diffusion or translation? In *Facilitating Technology Transfer through Partnership. Learning from Practice and Research*, ed. T. McMaster. Chapman and Hall.

Mead, Nicola, and Peter Bower. 2000. Patient-centredness: A conceptual framework and a review of the empirical literature. *Social Science & Medicine* 51 (7): 1087–1110.

Mesman, Jessica. 2007. Disturbing observations as a basis for collaborative research. *Science as Culture* 16 (3): 281–295.

Metzl, Jonathan A. 2010. Why against health? In *Against Health: How Health Became the New Morality*, ed. Jonathan A. Metzl and Anna Kirkland. New York University Press.

Metzl, Jonathan A., and Anna Kirkland, eds. 2010. *Against Health: How Health Became the New Morality*. New York University Press.

Ministry of Health Welfare and Sport. 2005. Better Faster. http: //www.snellerbeter. nl/english.

Mittman, Brian S. 2004. Creating the evidence base for quality improvement collaboratives. *Annals of Internal Medicine* 140 (11): 897–901.

Mol, Annemarie. 1999. Ontological politics; A word and some questions. In *Actor Network Theory and After*, ed. John Law and John Hassard. Blackwell.

Mol, Annemarie. 2002. *The Body Multiple: Ontology in Medical Practice*. Duke University Press.

Mol, Annemarie. 2008. *The Logic of Care: Health and the Problem of Patient Choice*. Routledge.

Moreira, Tiago. 2007. Entangled evidence: Knowledge making in systematic reviews in healthcare. *Sociology of Health & Illness* 29 (2): 180–197.

Mouffe, Chantal. 2000. *The Democratic Paradox*. Verso.

Mulkay, Michael, Jonathan Potter, and Steven Yearley. 1983. Why an analysis of scientific discourse is needed. In *Science Observed: Perspectives on the Social Study of Science*, ed. Karin Knorr Cetina and Michael Mulkay. SAGE.

Muniesa, Fabian, Yuval Millo, and Michel Callon. 2007. An introduction to market devices. In *Market Devices*, ed. Michel Callon, Yuval Millo, and Fabian Muniesa. Blackwell.

Murray, Mark, and Donald M. Berwick. 2003. Advanced access: Reducing waiting and delays in primary care. *Journal of the American Medical Association* 26 (8): 1035–1040.

Mykhalovskiy, Eric, and Lorna Weir. 2004. The problem of evidence-based medicine: Directions for social science. *Social Science & Medicine* 59 (5): 1059–1069.

Navaro, Vincent. 1976. *Medicine Under Capitalism*. Prodist.

Neuberger, Julia, C. Guthrie, and D. Aaronvitch. 2013. More care, less pathway: a review of the Liverpool Care Pathway. Department of Health, Crown Copyright.

Nickelsen, Niels Christian. 2009. Rethinking interventionist research: Navigating oppositional networks in a Danish hospital. *Journal of Research Practice* 5 (2): 1–18.

Nolan, T., R. Resar, C. Haraden, and F. A. Griffin. 2004. Improving the Reliability of Healthcare. IHI Innovation Series white paper, Institute for Healthcare Improvement.

Nowotny, Helga. 2007. How many policy rooms are there? Evidence-based and other kinds of science policies. *Science, Technology & Human Values* 32 (4): 479–490.

Oertle, Marc, and Roland Bal. 2010. Understanding non-adherence in chronic heart failure: A mixed-method case study. *Quality & Safety in Health Care* 19: 1–5.

Øvretveit, John. 2002. *Action Evaluation of Health Programmes and Change. A Handbook for a User-Focused Approach*. Radcliffe.

Øvretveit, J., P. Bate, P. Cleary, S. Cretin, D. Gustafson, K. McInnes, H. McLeod, et al. 2002. Quality collaboratives: Lessons from research. *Quality & Safety in Health Care* 11: 345–351.

Øvretveit, John, and D. Gustafson. 2002. Evaluation of quality improvement programmes. *Quality & Safety in Health Care* 11: 270–275.

Owens, Douglas K. 2011. Improving practice guidelines with patient-specific recommendations. *Annals of Internal Medicine* 154 (9): 638.

Palm, Ineke. 2005. *De zorg is geen markt: Een kritische analyse van de marktwerking in de zorg vanuit verschillende perspectieven*. Wetenschappelijk Bureau SP.

Parsons, Talcott. 1951. *The Social System*. Free Press.

Pasveer, Bernike. 1992. *Shadows of Knowledge—Making a Representing Practice in Medicine: X-Ray Pictures and Pulmonary Tuberculosis, 1895–1930*. University of Amsterdam.

Pinder, Ruth, Roland Petchey, Sara Shaw, and Yvonne Carter. 2005. What's in a care pathway? Towards a cultural cartography of the new NHS. *Sociology of Health & Illness* 27 (6): 759–779.

Platt, Tony. 1975. Prospects for a radical criminology. In *Critical Criminology*, ed. Ian Taylor, Paul Walton, and Jock Young. Routledge & Kegan Paul.

Pols, Jeanette. 2005. Enacting appreciations: Beyond the patient perspective. *Health Care Analysis* 13 (3): 203–221.

Polsky, Ned. 1967. Research method, morality and criminality. In Polsky, *Hustlers, Beats, and Others*. Aldine.

Porter, Michael E., and Elizabeth Olmsted Teisberg. 2004. Redefining competition in health care. *Harvard Business Review*, June: 65–76.

Porter, Theodore M. 1995. *Trust in Numbers: The Persuit of Objectivity in Science and Public Life*. Princeton University Press.

Porter, Theodore M. 1997. The management of society by numbers. In *Science in the Twentieth Century*, ed. John Krige and Dominique Pestre. Harwood.

Power, Michael. 1997. *The Audit Society. Rituals of Verification*. Oxford University Press.

Power, Michael. 2004. Counting, control and calculation: Reflections on measuring and management. *Human Relations* 57 (6): 765–783.

Prins, Baukje. 1995. The ethics of hybrid subjects: Feminist constructivism according to Donna Haraway. *Science, Technology & Human Values* 20 (3): 352–367.

Rainwater, Lee, and David J. Pittman. 1967. Ethical problems in studying a politically sensitive and deviant community. *Social Problems* 14 (4): 357–366.

Riley, Therese, Penelope Hawe, and Alan Shiell. 2005. Contested ground: How should qualitative evidence inform the conduct of a community intervention trial? *Journal of Health Services Research & Policy* 10 (2): 103–110.

Rip, Arie. 1986. Controversies as informal technology assessment. *Knowledge* 8 (2): 349–371.

Ritzer, George. 1992. *The McDonaldization of society. An investigation into the Changing Character of Contemporary Social Life.* Pine Forge.

Rodwin, Marc A. 1993. *Medicine, Money, and Morals: Physicians' Conflicts of Interest.* Oxford University Press.

Rogers, Everett M. 1962. *Diffusion of Innovations*, fourth edition (Free Press, 1995).

Roila, F. 2004. Transferring scientific evidence to oncological practice: A trial on the impact of three different implementation strategies on antiemetic prescriptions. *Supportive Care in Cancer* 12 (6): 446–453.

Rose, Hilary, and Steven Rose. 1969. *Science and Society.* Penguin.

Runciman, W. B. 2002. Lessons from the Australian Patient Safety Foundation: Setting up a national patient safety surveillance system. *Quality & Safety in Health Care* 11: 246–251.

Sackett, David L, and William M. C. Rosenberg. 1995. On the need for evidence-based medicine. *Journal of Public Health* 17 (3): 330–334.

Sackett, David L., William M. C. Rosenberg, J. A. Muir Gray, R. Brian Haynes, and W. Scott Richardson. 1996. Evidence based medicine: What it is and what it isn't. *British Medical Journal* 312 (7023): 71–72.

Sackett, David L, Sharon E. Straus, W. Scott Richardson, William M. C. Rosenberg, and R. Brian Haynes. 2000. *Evidence-Based Medicine: How to Practice and Teach EBM*, second edition. Churchgate Livingstone.

Scambler, Graham. 2008. *Sociology as Applied to Medicine*, sixth edition. Elsevier.

Schein, Edgar H. 1987. *Qualitative Research Methods*, volume 5: *The Clinical Perspective in Fieldwork.* SAGE.

Schouten, Loes M. T., Marlies E. J. Hulscher, Jannes J. E. van Everdingen, Robbert Huijsman, and Richard P. T. M. Grol. 2008. Evidence for the impact of quality improvement collaboratives: Systematic review. *British Medical Journal* 336: 1491–1494.

Schrijvers, Guus, Nico Oudendijk, and Pety de Vries. 2003. In search of the quickest way to disseminate health care innovations. *International Journal of Integrated Care* 3: 1–22.

Schut, Erik. 2003. *De zorg is toch geen markt? Laveren tussen marktfalen en overheidsfalen in de gezondheidszorg.* Oratiereeks Erasmus MC.

Schut, Erik. 2009. Is de marktwerking in de zorg doorgeschoten? *Socialisme & Democratie* 7/8: 68–80.

Scott, Pam, Evelleen Richards, and Brian Martin. 1990. Captives of controversy: The myth of the neutral social researcher in contemporary scientific controversies. *Science, Technology & Human Values* 15: 474–494.

Scriven, Michael 1991. *Evaluation Thesaurus*, fourth edition. SAGE.

Seeley, John R. 1967. The making and taking of problems: Toward an ethical stance. *Social Problems* 14 (4): 382–389.

Seifer, Sarena. D. 2010. *Handbook of Engaged Scholarship: Contemporary Landscapes, Future Directions*, volume 1: *Institutional Change*. Michigan State University Press.

Sellen, Abigail J., and Richard H. R. Harper. 2002. *The Myth of the Paperless Office.* MIT Press.

Senge, Peter, and C. Otto Scharmer. 2001. Community action research. In *The SAGE Handbook of Action Research*, ed. Peter Reason and Hilary Bradbury. SAGE.

Shapin, Steven, and Simon Schaffer. 1985. *Leviathan and the Air-Pump: Hobbes, Boyle, and the Experimental Life*. Princeton University Press.

Shell Nederland. 2004. *Here You Work Safely or You Don't Work Here at All.* Shell Nederland.

Silverman, David. 1987. *Communication and Medical Practice: Social Relations in the Clinic.* SAGE.

Silvester, Kate, Richard Lendon, Helen Bevan, Richard Steyn, and Paul Walley. 2004. Reducing waiting times in the NHS: Is lack of capacity the problem? *Clinician in Management* 12: 105–111.

Simborg, D. 1981. DRG creep: A new hospital-acquired disease. *New England Journal of Medicine* 304 (26): 1602–1604.

Sjögren, Ebba, and Claes-Frederik Helgesson. 2007. The Q(u)ALYfying hand: Health economics and medicine in the shaping of Swedish markets for subsidized pharmaceuticals. In *Market Devices*, ed. Michel Callon, Yuval Millo, and Fabian Muniesa. Blackwell.

Smith, Adam. 1776. *The Wealth of Nations*, volume I (Modern Library, 2000).

Smith, Matthew. 2011. Second opinions: Mixing with medics. *Social History of Medicine* 24 (1): 142–150.

Star, Susan Leigh. 1991a. Invisible work and silenced dialogues in knowledge representation. In *Women, Work and Computerization*, ed. Inger V. Eriksson, B. A. Kitchenham and Kea Tijdens. Elsevier.

Star, Susan Leigh. 1991b. Power, technology and the phenomenology of conventions: On being allergic to onions. In *A Sociology of Monsters: Essays on Power, Technology and Domination*, ed. John Law. Routledge.

Star, Susan Leigh, ed. 1995. *Ecologies of Knowledge: Work and Politics in Science and Technology*. State University of New York Press.

Star, Susan Leigh, and Anselm Strauss. 1999. Layers of silence, arenas of voice: The ecology of visible and invisible work. *Computer Supported Cooperative Work* 8: 9–30.

Steen Carlsson, K., S. Hojgard, A. Glomstein, S. Lethagen, S. Schulman, L. Tengborn, A. Lindgren, E. Berntorp, and B. Lindgren. 2003. On-demand vs. prophylactic treatment for severe haemophilia in Norway and Sweden: Differences in treatment characteristics and outcome. *Haemophilia* 9 (5): 555–566.

Steinbusch, Paul, Jan Oostenbrink, Joost Zuurbier, and J. Schaepkens. 2007. The risk of upcoding in casemix systems: A comparative study. *Health Policy* 81: 289–299.

Stewart, M., J. Brown, W. Weston, I. McWhinney, C. McWilliam, and T. Freeman. 1995. *Patient-Centred Medicine: Transforming the Clinical Method*. SAGE.

Stinchcombe, Arthur L. 2007. Speaking truth to the public, and indirectly to power. In *Public Sociology: Fifteen Eminent Sociologists Debate the Politics and the Profession in the Twenty-First Century*, ed. Dan Clawson, Robert Zussman, Joya Misra, Naomi Gerstel, Randall Stokes, Douglas L. Anderton, and Michael Burawoy. University of California Press.

Strathern, Marilyn. 1991. *Partial Connections*. Rowman & Littlefield.

Strathern, Marilyn. 1992. The decomposition of an event. *Cultural Anthropology* 7: 244–254.

Straus, Robert. 1957. The nature and status of medical sociology. *American Sociological Review* 22 (2): 200–204.

Straus, Robert. 1999. Medical sociology: A personal fifty year perspective. *Journal of Health and Social Behavior* 40 (2): 103–110.

Strauss, Anselm L. 1978. A social world perspective. *Studies in Symbolic Interaction* 1: 119–128.

Strauss, Anselm, Shizuko Fagerhaugh, Barbara Suczek, and Carolyn Wiener. 1997. *Social Organization of Medical Work*. Transaction.

Stroke Prevention in Atrial Fibrillation Investigators. 1991. Stroke prevention in atrial fibrillation study: Final results. *Circulation* 84 (2): 527–539.

Suchman, Lucy. 1987. *Plans and Situated Actions: The Problem of Human-Machine Communication.* Cambridge University Press.

Suchman, Lucy. 1995. Representations of work: Making work visible. *Communications of the ACM* 38 (9): 56–64.

Suchman, Lucy. 2000. Making a case: "Knowledge" and "routine" work in knowledge production. In *Workplace Studies: Recovering Work Practice and Informing System Design*, ed. Paul Luff, Jon Hindmarsh, and Christian Heath. Cambridge University Press.

Suchman, Lucy. 2002. Located accountabilities in technology production. *Scandinavian Journal of Information Systems* 14 (2): 91–105.

Suchman, Lucy. 2007. *Human-Machine Reconfigurations: Plans and Situated Actions,* second edition. Cambridge University Press.

Suchman, Lucy. 2008. Feminist STS and the sciences of the artificial. In *The Handbook of Science and Technology Studies*, ed. Edward J. Hackett, Olga Amsterdamska, Michael Lynch, and Judy Wajcman. MIT Press.

Suchman, Lucy, and Randall Trigg. 1991. Understanding practice: Video as a medium for reflection and design. In *Design at Work: Cooperative Design of Computer Systems*, ed. Joan Greenbaum and Morten Kyng. Erlbaum.

Tanenbaum, Sandra J. 1994. Knowing and acting in medical practice: The epistemological politics of outcomes research. *Journal of Health Politics, Policy and Law* 19 (1): 27–44.

Tanenbaum, Sandra J. 2005. Evidence-based practice as mental health policy: Three controversies and a caveat. *Health Affairs* 24 (1): 163–174.

Tarde, Gabriel. 1902. *Psychologie Èconomique.* Félix Alcan.

Taylor, E., and J. Z. Taylor. 2004. Using qualitative psychology to investigate HACCP implementation barriers. *International Journal of Environmental Health Research* 14 (1): 53–63.

The, Anne-Mei. 1999. *Palliatieve behandeling en communicatie een onderzoek naar het optimisme op herstel van longkankerpatiënten.* Bohn Stafleu Van Loghum.

The, Anne-Mei, Tony Hak, Gerard Koëter, and Gerrit van der Wal. 2000. Collusion in doctor-patient communication about imminent death: An ethnographic study. *British Medical Journal* 321: 1376–1381.

Thévenot, Laurent. 1984. Rules and implements: Investment in forms. *Social Sciences Information. Information Sur les Sciences Sociales* 23 (1): 1–45.

Thévenot, Laurent. 1993. Essai sur les objets usuels. In *Les objets dans l'action: De la maison au laboratoire*, ed. Bernard Conein, Nicolas Dodier, and Laurent Thévenot. École des Hautes Études en Sciences Sociales.

Thévenot, Laurent. 2001. Organized complexity: Conventions of coordination and the composition of economic arrangements. *European Journal of Social Theory* 4 (4): 405–425.

Thévenot, Laurent. 2002. Which road to follow? The moral complexity of an "equipped" humanity. In *Complexities: Social Studies of Knowledge Practices*, ed. John Law and Annemarie Mol. Duke University Press.

Thomas, William Isaac. 1914. The Polish-Prussian situation: An experiment in assimilation. *American Journal of Sociology* 19 (5): 624–639.

Timmermans, Stefan. 2010. Evidence-based medicine: Sociological explorations. In *Handbook of Medical Sociology*, sixth edition, ed. Chloe E. Bird, Peter Conrad, Allen M. Fremont, and Stefan Timmermans. Vanderbilt University Press.

Timmermans, Stefan, and Marc Berg. 2003. *The Gold Standard: The Challenge of Evidence-Based Medicine and Standardization in Health Care*. Temple University Press.

Timmermans, Stefan, and Steven Haas. 2008. Towards a sociology of disease. *Sociology of Health & Illness* 30 (5): 659–676.

Timmermans, Stefan, and Aaron Mauck. 2005. The promises and pitfalls of evidence-based medicine. *Health Affairs* 24 (1): 18–29.

Tittle, Charles R. 2004. The arrogance of public sociology. *Social Forces* 82 (4): 1639–1643.

TPG. 2004. Het kan écht: Betere zorg voor minder geld.

Traore, A. N., A. K. C. Chan, K. E. Webert, N. Heddle, B. Ritchie, J. St-Louis, J. Teitel, D. Lillicrap, A. Iorio, and I. Walker. 2014. First analysis of 10-year trends in national factor concentrates usage in haemophilia: Data from CHARMS, the Canadian Hemophilia Assessment and Resource Management System. *Haemophilia* 20 (4): e251–e259.

van der Lei, Johan. 1991. Use and abuse of computer-stored medical records. *Methods of Information in Medicine* 30: 79–80.

van der Ploeg, Irma. 2001. *Prosthetic Bodies. The Construction of the Fetus and the Couple as Patients in Reproductive Technologies*. Kluwer.

van de Ven, Andrew H. 2007. *Engaged Scholarship: A Guide for Organizational and Social Research*. Oxford University Press.

van Egmond, Stans, and Teun Zuiderent-Jerak. 2010. Analysing policy change: The performative role of economics in the constitution of a new policy programme in

Dutch health care. In *Science and Policy in Interaction: On Practices of Science Policy Interactions for Policy-Making in Health Care*, ed. Stans van Egmond. Erasmus University.

van Geenen, Ronald. 2005. Aanval op medische missers. *Algemeen Dagblad*, November 24.

Vanhaecht, K., and W. Sermeus. 2002. Draaiboek voor de ontwikkeling, implementatie en evaluatie van een klinisch pad: 30 stappenplan van het netwerk klinische paden. *Acta Hospitalia* 3: 13–27.

van Loon, Ester, and Teun Zuiderent-Jerak. 2012. Framing reflexivity in quality improvement devices in the care for older people. *Health Care Analysis* 20 (2): 119–138.

Verran, Helen. 2001. *Science and an African Logic*. University of Chicago Press.

Verran, Helen. 2012. *Numbers and Nature. Lecture given at the WTMC Summer School: Seeing Through Numbers*. Ravenstein.

Vikkelsø, Signe. 2007. Description, resistance, and intervention. *Science as Culture* 16 (3): 297–309.

Wachelder, Joseph. 2003. Democratizing science: Various routes and visions of Dutch science shops. *Science, Technology & Human Values* 28 (2): 244–273.

Wagner, Ina. 1993. Women's voice: The case of nursing information systems. *AI & Society* 7: 295–310.

Waitzkin, Howard. 1983. *The Second Sickness: Contradictions of Capitalist Health Care*. Free Press.

Watson-Verran, Helen, and David Turnbull. 1995. Science and other indigenous knowledge systems. In *Handbook of Science and Technology Studies*, ed. Sheila Jasanoff, Gerald E. Markle, James C. Petersen, and Trevor Pinch. SAGE.

Weber, Max. 1918–19. Science as a vocation. In *From Max Weber: Essays in Sociology*, ed. H. Gerth and C. W. Mills (Oxford University Press, 1991).

Webster, Andrew. 2007a. Crossing boundaries: Social science in the policy room. *Science, Technology & Human Values* 32 (4): 458–478.

Webster, Andrew. 2007b. Reflections on reflexive engagement: Response to Nowotny and Wynne. *Science, Technology & Human Values* 32 (5): 608–615.

Weisz, George, Alberto Cambrosio, Peter Keating, Loes Knaapen, Thomas Schlich, and Virginie J. Tournay. 2007. The emergence of clinical practice guidelines. *Milbank Quarterly* 85 (4): 691–727.

Wennberg, John E. 1984. Dealing with medical practice variations: A proposal for action. *Health Affairs* 3 (2): 6–32.

Wennberg, John E., and M. M. Cooper. 1999. *The Quality of Medical Care in the United States: A Report on the Medicare Program*. American Hospital Publishing.

Wennberg, John E., and Alan Gittelsohn. 1973. Small area variations in health care delivery. *Science* 183: 1102–1108.

Wensing, Michel, Hub Wollersheim, and Richard Grol. 2006. Organizational interventions to implement improvements in patient care: A structured review of reviews. *Implementation Science* 1 (2): 1–9.

White, Joseph. 1991. *Competitive Solutions: American Health Care Proposals and International Experience*. Brookings Institution.

Willems, Dick. 1995. Tools of Care: Explorations into the Semiotics of Medical Technology. PhD dissertation, University of Maastricht.

Willems, Dick. 2000. Managing one's body using self-management techniques: Practicing autonomy. *Theoretical Medicine and Bioethics* 21: 23–38.

Willems, Dick. 2001. Dokters en patiënten in kleine medische technologie. In *Ingebouwde normen, medische technieken doorgelicht*, ed. Marc Berg and Annemarie Mol. Van der Wees.

Williams, Bernard. 1985. *Ethics and the Limits of Philosophy* (Routledge, 2011).

Willmore, Douglas W., and Henrik Kehlet. 2001. Management of patients in fast track surgery. *British Medical Journal* 322 (7284): 473–476.

Winthereik, Brit Ross, Antoinette de Bont, and Marc Berg. 2002. Assessing the world of doctors and their computers: "Making available" objects of study and the researh site through ethnographic engagement. *Scandinavian Journal of Information Systems* 14 (2): 47–58.

Woodhouse, Edward, David Hess, Steve Breyman, and Brian Martin. 2002. Science studies and activism: Possibilities and problems for reconstructivist agendas. *Social Studies of Science* 32 (2): 297–319.

Woolgar, Steve. 1983. Irony in the social studies of science. In *Science Observed*, ed. Karin Knorr Cetina and Michael Mulkay. SAGE.

Woolgar, Steve. 1991. The turn to technology in social studies of science. *Science, Technology & Human Values* 16 (1): 20–50.

Woolgar, Steve, and Javier Lezaun. 2013. The wrong bin bag: A turn to ontology in science and technology studies? *Social Studies of Science* 43 (3): 321–340.

Wynne, Brian. 2007. Dazzled by the mirage of influence? STS-SSK in multivalent registers of relevance. *Science, Technology & Human Values* 32 (4): 491–503.

ZonMw. 2008. Patient safety. http://www.zonmw.nl/en/programmes/all-programmes/patient-safety/.

Zuiderent, Teun. 2002. Blurring the center: On the politics of ethnography. *Scandinavian Journal of Information Systems* 14 (2): 59–78.

Zuiderent, Teun, Brit Ross Winthereik, and Marc Berg. 2003. Talking about distributed communication and medicine: On bringing together remote and local actors. *Human-Computer Interaction* 18 (1): 171–180.

Zuiderent-Jerak, Teun. 2007. Preventing implementation: Experimental interventions with standardization in healthcare. *Science as Culture* 16 (3): 311–329.

Zuiderent-Jerak, Teun. 2009. Competition in the wild: Configuring healthcare markets. *Social Studies of Science* 39 (5): 765–792.

Zuiderent-Jerak, Teun. 2010. Embodied interventions—interventions on bodies: Experiments in practices of science and technology studies and hemophilia care. *Science, Technology & Human Values* 35 (5): 677–710.

Zuiderent-Jerak, Teun, and Casper Bruun Jensen. 2007. Unpacking 'intervention' in Science and Technology Studies. *Science as Culture* 16 (3): 227–235.

Zuiderent-Jerak, Teun, Roland Bal, and Marc Berg. 2012. Patients and their problems: Situated alliances of patient-centred care and pathway development. In *Cancer Patients, Cancer Pathways: Historical and Sociological Perspectives*, ed. Carsten Timmermann and Elizabeth Toon. Palgrave Macmillan.

Zuiderent-Jerak, Teun, Frode Forland, and Fergus Macbeth. 2012. Guidelines should reflect all knowledge, not just clinical trials. *British Medical Journal* 345 (e6702).

Zuiderent-Jerak, Teun, Mathilde Strating, Anna Nieboer, and Roland Bal. 2009. Sociological refigurations of patient safety: Ontologies of improvement and "acting with" quality collaboratives in healthcare. *Social Science & Medicine* 69 (12): 1713–1721.

Zuiderent-Jerak, Teun, Kor Grit, and Tom van der Grinten. 2015. Critical composition of public values: On the enactment and disarticulation of what counts in healthcare markets. In *Value Practices in the Life Sciences and Medicine*, ed. Claes-Frederik Helgesson, Francis Lee, and Isabelle Dussauge. Oxford University Press.

Index

Inside Technology

edited by Wiebe E. Bijker, W. Bernard Carlson, and Trevor Pinch

Teun Zuiderent-Jerak, *Situated Intervention: Sociological Experiments in Health Care*

Basile Zimmermann, *Technology and Cultural Difference: Electronic Music Devices, Social Networking Sites, and Computer Encodings in Contemporary China*

Andrew J. Nelson, *The Sound of Innovation: Stanford and the Computer Music Revolution*

Sonja D. Schmid, *Producing Power: The Pre-Chernobyl History of the Soviet Nuclear Industry*

Casey O'Donnell, *Developer's Dilemma: The Secret World of Videogame Creators*

Christina Dunbar-Hester, *Low Power to the People: Pirates, Protest, and Politics in FM Radio Activism*

Eden Medina, Ivan da Costa Marques, and Christina Holmes, editors, *Beyond Imported Magic: Essays on Science, Technology, and Society in Latin America*

Anique Hommels, Jessica Mesman, and Wiebe E. Bijker, editors, *Vulnerability in Technological Cultures: New Directions in Research and Governance*

Amit Prasad, *Imperial Technoscience: Transnational Histories of MRI in the United States, Britain, and India*

Charis Thompson, *Good Science: The Ethical Choreography of Stem Cell Research*

Tarleton Gillespie, Pablo J. Boczkowski, and Kirsten A. Foot, editors, *Media Technologies: Essays on Communication, Materiality, and Society*

Catelijne Coopmans, Janet Vertesi, Michael Lynch, and Steve Woolgar, editors, *Representation in Scientific Practice Revisited*

Rebecca Slayton, *Arguments that Count: Physics, Computing, and Missile Defense, 1949–2012*

Stathis Arapostathis and Graeme Gooday, *Patently Contestable: Electrical Technologies and Inventor Identities on Trial in Britain*

Jens Lachmund, *Greening Berlin: The Co-Production of Science, Politics, and Urban Nature*

Chikako Takeshita, *The Global Biopolitics of the IUD: How Science Constructs Contraceptive Users and Women's Bodies*

Cyrus C. M. Mody, *Instrumental Community: Probe Microscopy and the Path to Nanotechnology*

Morana Alač, *Handling Digital Brains: A Laboratory Study of Multimodal Semiotic Interaction in the Age of Computers*

Gabrielle Hecht, editor, *Entangled Geographies: Empire and Technopolitics in the Global Cold War*

Michael E. Gorman, editor, *Trading Zones and Interactional Expertise: Creating New Kinds of Collaboration*

Matthias Gross, *Ignorance and Surprise: Science, Society, and Ecological Design*

Andrew Feenberg, *Between Reason and Experience: Essays in Technology and Modernity*

Wiebe E. Bijker, Roland Bal, and Ruud Hendricks, *The Paradox of Scientific Authority: The Role of Scientific Advice in Democracies*

Park Doing, *Velvet Revolution at the Synchrotron: Biology, Physics, and Change in Science*

Gabrielle Hecht, *The Radiance of France: Nuclear Power and National Identity after World War II*

Richard Rottenburg, *Far-Fetched Facts: A Parable of Development Aid*

Michel Callon, Pierre Lascoumes, and Yannick Barthe, *Acting in an Uncertain World: An Essay on Technical Democracy*

Ruth Oldenziel and Karin Zachmann, editors, *Cold War Kitchen: Americanization, Technology, and European Users*

Deborah G. Johnson and Jameson W. Wetmore, editors, *Technology and Society: Building Our Sociotechnical Future*

Trevor Pinch and Richard Swedberg, editors, *Living in a Material World: Economic Sociology Meets Science and Technology Studies*

Christopher R. Henke, *Cultivating Science, Harvesting Power: Science and Industrial Agriculture in California*

Helga Nowotny, *Insatiable Curiosity: Innovation in a Fragile Future*

Karin Bijsterveld, *Mechanical Sound: Technology, Culture, and Public Problems of Noise in the Twentieth Century*

Peter D. Norton, *Fighting Traffic: The Dawn of the Motor Age in the American City*

Joshua M. Greenberg, *From Betamax to Blockbuster: Video Stores and the Invention of Movies on Video*

Mikael Hård and Thomas J. Misa, editors, *Urban Machinery: Inside Modern European Cities*

Christine Hine, *Systematics as Cyberscience: Computers, Change, and Continuity in Science*

Wesley Shrum, Joel Genuth, and Ivan Chompalov, *Structures of Scientific Collaboration*

Shobita Parthasarathy, *Building Genetic Medicine: Breast Cancer, Technology, and the Comparative Politics of Health Care*

Kristen Haring, *Ham Radio's Technical Culture*

Atsushi Akera, *Calculating a Natural World: Scientists, Engineers and Computers during the Rise of U.S. Cold War Research*

Donald MacKenzie, *An Engine, Not a Camera: How Financial Models Shape Markets*

Geoffrey C. Bowker, *Memory Practices in the Sciences*

Christophe Lécuyer, *Making Silicon Valley: Innovation and the Growth of High Tech, 1930–1970*

Anique Hommels, *Unbuilding Cities: Obduracy in Urban Sociotechnical Change*

David Kaiser, editor, *Pedagogy and the Practice of Science: Historical and Contemporary Perspectives*

Charis Thompson, *Making Parents: The Ontological Choreography of Reproductive Technology*

Pablo J. Boczkowski, *Digitizing the News: Innovation in Online Newspapers*

Dominique Vinck, editor, *Everyday Engineering: An Ethnography of Design and Innovation*

Nelly Oudshoorn and Trevor Pinch, editors, *How Users Matter: The Co-Construction of Users and Technology*

Peter Keating and Alberto Cambrosio, *Biomedical Platforms: Realigning the Normal and the Pathological in Late-Twentieth-Century Medicine*

Paul Rosen, *Framing Production: Technology, Culture, and Change in the British Bicycle Industry*

Maggie Mort, *Building the Trident Network: A Study of the Enrollment of People, Knowledge, and Machines*

Donald MacKenzie, *Mechanizing Proof: Computing, Risk, and Trust*

Geoffrey C. Bowker and Susan Leigh Star, *Sorting Things Out: Classification and Its Consequences*

Charles Bazerman, *The Languages of Edison's Light*

Janet Abbate, *Inventing the Internet*

Herbert Gottweis, *Governing Molecules: The Discursive Politics of Genetic Engineering in Europe and the United States*

Kathryn Henderson, *On Line and On Paper: Visual Representation, Visual Culture, and Computer Graphics in Design Engineering*

Susanne K. Schmidt and Raymund Werle, *Coordinating Technology: Studies in the International Standardization of Telecommunications*

Marc Berg, *Rationalizing Medical Work: Decision Support Techniques and Medical Practices*

Eda Kranakis, *Constructing a Bridge: An Exploration of Engineering Culture, Design, and Research in Nineteenth-Century France and America*

Paul N. Edwards, *The Closed World: Computers and the Politics of Discourse in Cold War America*

Donald MacKenzie, *Knowing Machines: Essays on Technical Change*

Wiebe E. Bijker, *Of Bicycles, Bakelites, and Bulbs: Toward a Theory of Sociotechnical Change*

Louis L. Bucciarelli, *Designing Engineers*

Geoffrey C. Bowker, *Science on the Run: Information Management and Industrial Geophysics at Schlumberger, 1920–1940*

Wiebe E. Bijker and John Law, editors, *Shaping Technology / Building Society: Studies in Sociotechnical Change*

Stuart Blume, *Insight and Industry: On the Dynamics of Technological Change in Medicine*

Donald MacKenzie, *Inventing Accuracy: A Historical Sociology of Nuclear Missile Guidance*

Pamela E. Mack, *Viewing the Earth: The Social Construction of the Landsat Satellite System*

H. M. Collins, *Artificial Experts: Social Knowledge and Intelligent Machines*

http://mitpress.mit.edu/books/series/inside-technology